HOW
WAR
KILLS

HOW WAR KILLS

YARA M. ASI, PhD

THE OVERLOOKED THREATS TO OUR HEALTH

JOHNS HOPKINS UNIVERSITY PRESS | *Baltimore*

© 2024 Johns Hopkins University Press
All rights reserved. Published 2024
Printed in the United States of America on acid-free paper
9 8 7 6 5 4 3 2 1

Johns Hopkins University Press
2715 North Charles Street
Baltimore, Maryland 21218
www.press.jhu.edu

Library of Congress Cataloging-in-Publication Data is available.

ISBN 978-1-4214-4789-6 (paperback)
ISBN 978-1-4214-4790-2 (ebook)

A catalog record for this book is available from the British Library.

Special discounts are available for bulk purchases of this book. For more information, please contact Special Sales at specialsales@jh.edu.

To Brett, Z, and Ash
FOR YOUR LOVE

To Alia
FOR YOUR STRENGTH

To Morad
FOR YOUR WORDS

CONTENTS

ACKNOWLEDGMENTS

IT IS HARD TO ACKNOWLEDGE all the things that had to happen for this book to exist, many of which I had nothing to do with. My mother had no precedent for being an independent person who ignored the norms that were expected of women of her place and time. She continued to overcome unimaginable obstacles in her life while still ensuring that I had the opportunity to have the life I imagined for myself. She has supported me every step of the way and is always my biggest fan. Out of necessity, when I was very young, she would often bring me with her when she went to campus as she was pursuing her graduate degree. I hung around her and other graduate students, understanding little that they said but loving the vibe of sitting around in a computer lab, talking about cool ideas with others, and getting excited about possibilities. It planted the seed for who I would eventually become. Mom, all of this is for you.

I wish I could have shared this book with my dad. His influence, too, is incalculable, despite my having little time with him. His short presence in my life taught me how random all of this is and how, really, nothing is more important than our health and the health and well-being of the people we love. As I was writing this book, I felt my dad's presence with every word I wrote. I think he'd really like it.

I would not be the person I am today without the experiences I have heard about, witnessed, and experienced in Palestine. I am beyond grateful to be from such a beautiful place that has taught me so much about what life is truly about. Far from just being some setting of war, political failure, trauma, and injustice, Palestine is my grandmother's hands kneading dough, picking figs with my cousins, eating gooey knafeh at one in the morning, and the earthy smell of freshly pressed olive oil. (Is it clear enough how much I miss the food there?) I especially want to acknowledge my uncle Fayez, who unfortunately passed away before this book was published. He was a father figure to me who went above and beyond to support our family, and I miss him dearly. And of course, my other uncle, whose story I share at the beginning of the book. Seeing how his experience affected our family was truly life changing, and I am so grateful he is still here, tending to his olive and pomegranate trees.

Most of this book was written during the height of the pandemic, through lockdowns and school closures and a lot of stress and uncertainty. It would have been impossible to do this without the support of my husband, Brett. And I want to acknowledge my two amazing sons, who served as my inspiration for this and for everything else. I want to help create a better world for them. I hope this book furthers that goal.

I have been so lucky to have such great friends who provided support throughout the long process of researching and writing the book (with helpful questions like "When is your book coming out?" and "Why is your book taking so long?"). One friend went out of his way by being the only person, aside from me, to read every word of this book before it was submitted and who provided me with pages of helpful—and honest—comments. He also responded to many completely out-of-the-blue texts about word choice and grammar without flinching. (I highly recommend having an editor as a best friend.) Nathan, thank you so much for making me feel like maybe this could be a decent book in the end.

I also want to thank my other friends and loved ones whose support was invaluable as I was writing the book: Charles, Adam, Ahmed, Kristen, Ana, Ellen, my colleagues at the University of Central Florida, and my fellow codirectors of the Palestine Program for Health and Human Rights. Thank you also to Christian Davenport for reading early chapters of the book and offering some great suggestions for the title. And I could not forget the dear people I have met through the American Public Health Association, especially through the Peace Caucus and the Primary Prevention of War Working Group; when I joined APHA as a graduate student, I was still not sure whether I could dedicate my career to studying the health of people in war. Through APHA, I met many of the people already doing that hard work, who had written so many of the books and articles that were foundational to my own intellectual development. Their formal and informal support has been invaluable. A special thank you to Amy Hagopian, whom I interviewed for this book and whom I feel fortunate to consider now a friend.

This book certainly wouldn't have happened if my colleague Dr. Basia Andraka-Christou had not introduced me to her (and now my) editor, Robin Coleman. Basia, thank you for helping me believe this was possible and for answering my many, many, possibly too many, questions about the process. Robin, thank you for helping me turn that tiny sliver of hope into a reality. Thank you to everyone I worked with at Johns Hopkins University Press, including the anonymous peer reviewers, for their support of this book and to the great editors at Inksplash who read it with such care to make it the best book it could be.

INTRODUCTION

I'll pay no heed to what's happening outside the window—shells, rockets, ships, jets, artillery—all blowing my way like a raging wind, falling like rain, shaking the place like an earthquake. Human will can't do anything against these; they're a fate that can't be turned back. All the unimaginably evil inventions human creativity has ever come up with and all the advances technology has achieved— their efficacy is now being tested on our bodies.

—MAHMOUD DARWISH,
Memory for Forgetfulness: August, Beirut, 1982 (1995)

BY 2030, ABOUT HALF of the people living in extreme poverty around the world will live in a territory that is experiencing conflict (World Bank, 2016). Social media has ensured that, from the comfort of your kitchen in Hamburg or Miami or Sydney, you can see the most horrific images of war in ways we never have before: a young boy's body washed up on the beach; an emaciated infant girl suffering from famine; a shell-shocked child sitting in an ambulance, face still matted with dirt and blood from the attack he survived.

Although these images are real representations of war, they can obscure other effects of war that are not as visibly traumatic. It is natural to see such physical trauma and feel moved by its presence. It is much more difficult to relate to the trauma of, for example, a statistical model showing a country losing its access to safe drinking water because of conflict-related actions. If we even happen to come across such a story, we feel sad, frustrated, even sympathetic—but these stories do not tend to go viral, and they rarely seem to drive policy decisions. As a result, so many things that we could do to make life better for so many people are not being prioritized.

Let me tell you a story about my family.

Ibrahim was, unmistakably, the family patriarch in a society where that still meant something. (I changed his name here to protect his privacy.) He knew everyone, he was quick and persuasive, and he knew how to get things done. In the West Bank, one of the two territories that make up the occupied Palestinian territories, knowing how to get things done has always been a vital skill for success. His father had died decades before, but even when his father was alive, Ibrahim was the son who went abroad to study, living first in France and then in the United States. Ibrahim was the one who pushed his father to allow his younger sister to be able to attend college in a different country—unheard of for women at the time. Ibrahim was a highly respected college professor, then a college administrator, and even briefly worked in government, in the education ministry. He had been married for decades to a successful architect, raising five children in an apartment building that his wife had designed. He could not walk down the streets of the city without hearing greetings from colleagues, friends, or former students. By all accounts, Ibrahim was a success story in an environment where success was by no means guaranteed.

That sister whom Ibrahim had pushed to go to college abroad so many years before—my mother—was now sitting on her bed almost 7,000 miles away, crying. "How can this be happening?" she asked, distraught. "Not Ibrahim. No." I asked her if she knew what was wrong. She said that he had been feeling weak for a few days and then had suddenly collapsed. A stroke? A heart attack? "They don't think so," she told me. "Guillain-Barré syndrome. Do you know what that is? Do you know anything about it? What is it?"

I had just finished a master's program and had been planning to go to medical school or maybe train to be a physician's assistant, but I had never heard of Guillain-Barré. I googled it on my phone. It sounded bad, but I noted the words *treatable* and *full recovery*. I held up the phone for my mother, willing her to read the information through her tears. "It's okay, Mom, it's treatable."

She *tsk*ed, and said, in a tone I recognized immediately, "*Mush fi Falastin.*" Not in Palestine.

Today, more than a decade later, my uncle is fine. The patriarch lives on. Yet my mother was right: he wasn't going to get healthy in Palestine. Without the special permits he obtained to enter a hospital in Israel, he might not have recovered. Had my uncle stayed in France or the United States, he would likely have undergone a scary, but short-lived, period of diagnosis and treatment. He wasn't from an elite or rich lineage; he grew up in a one-room stone home, sleeping on the floor with his two brothers, three sisters (including my mother), and their parents. They washed their own clothes by hand and chased down the chickens they planned to eat on the one or two days a week they could afford meat. Like so many born into an unforgiving environment, my uncle went abroad to pursue his education. But to build a life, he eventually chose to move back to a place that had been experiencing violence, restriction, and deprivation for his whole life. He does not think he will live long enough to see it get any better.

When my uncle fell ill, I of course knew that my home country was technically undergoing what most people called conflict, although fortunately there weren't many active bombing campaigns in the West Bank anymore. I'd written several papers about it for school history fairs—even making it to the county history fair once—and gotten raised eyebrows from several teachers when I proudly presented my middle-school mind's understanding of what was, even then, one of the longest and most polarizing settings of armed conflict in modern times.

We went back to the West Bank regularly during summer breaks, in true diaspora fashion. I'd been stopped on the street by soldiers and questioned during my visits; border agents had leafed through my *Baby-Sitters Club* books, tucked carefully into my pink "Going to Grandma's" suitcase. (This was pre-iPad and before planes had installed an individual TV for every seat—you needed a lot of books for that plane ride.) I'd been stopped at countless checkpoints, been questioned by hostile soldiers holding rifles, seen military jeeps racing through the streets of my grandmother's village. From these occasional experiences, I thought I knew what war could look like.

In the early 2000s, during the second *Intifada* (Arabic for "uprising"), we took a few years off from visiting. Even then, I didn't fully understand why. Each summer during that period, I'd ask my mother if we were going. She'd *tsk* in that way of hers: "It's bad there right now." That was usually the end of the conversation.

This book is my effort to capture the multifaceted effects of war and conflict on the health of civilian populations, focusing on contemporary conflicts but also drawing from recent and distant history to help us understand how we got to this moment. What I've learned in the years since I was a child—split between what seemed like two different planets—is that war is the greatest threat to human health and well-being, even in places where the wars themselves are not fought.

The most obvious effects of war on health arise from what we might refer to as direct violence: bombing, shooting, kidnapping, torture, and so on. In addition to this direct violence, I highlight the structural barriers to health that are almost purely political: the physical or administrative blocking of the movement of patients, providers, or medical goods; the inability of civilians to secure nutritious food or engage in healthy behaviors; and the heightened risk of infectious disease as vulnerable populations cluster or move into new areas.

For conflict-affected populations, war is the ultimate determinant of health. Yet even in developed and mostly peaceful societies, overly militarized perspectives on defense and security have shifted trillions of dollars toward maintaining and expanding a military presence. These funds could instead be used to fill gaps in housing, food and water security, education, and direct health services. As long as the relationship of health to war is one of response—that is, ministering to physical or mental trauma only after the fact—we will miss out on the potential of health care and health system stakeholders to not only prevent war, but reduce human suffering more broadly.

CONFLICT: THE ULTIMATE SOCIAL DETERMINANT OF HEALTH

Ibrahim is now mostly retired. He's healthy, or as healthy as a 70ish-year-old man can be. He bought some farmland on a mountain, and he loves to go there and inspect his bounty: pomegranate and fig trees teeming with fruit, grapevines delicately strung from overhead lattices, and a lone prickly pear cactus he planted near a wall so as to avoid accidentally brushing against its spines. His children are getting married and having their own children. His eldest son has taken up his mantle, gently assuming his father's role of getting things done for neighbors, dealing with family matters, and being the one who is high-fived on the street by seemingly everyone. Ibrahim hopes his health problems are over, at least for now. His journey back to health, across borders, was exhausting for him and his family; he doesn't want to put anyone through that again. Living in an area of conflict, however, is one of the most insidious social determinants of health. It reaches into every aspect of your life: where you live, how you make your money, whom you can marry, the food you can eat, and the safety of your children.

Recently, Ibrahim's youngest daughter was having issues with one of her eyes. She went to various eye doctors, and it was ultimately decided that she needed an operation, one that she could not receive in the West Bank. Fortunately, her family had enough money to send her to Jordan for the operation at a private facility. Jordan's demographics are relatively similar to those of the West Bank. They share a religion, a culture, and a language, and Amman, Jordan's capital, is less than 50 miles from Nablus in the West Bank. Yet a trip into Jordan, for any reason, requires citizenship paperwork, transportation to a border crossing, and an hours-long wait in a series of lines and security checkpoints staffed by armed soldiers. Nevertheless, thousands of Palestinians cross the border every year—to Jordan, Egypt, and even Israel—for medical care they can't receive in their own country. *Mush fi Falastin*. Not in Palestine.

My uncle's experience is by no means the standard for a civilian seeking health care in an area suffering from war or political violence, as he was struck by a condition that afflicts less than 40 people per million.

Rather than experience such a rare ailment, the average person in a conflict-affected area is far more likely to have inadequate access to basic primary care, maternity care, vaccinations, food, water, or sanitation. The situation in the West Bank is unique, and every setting of war has its own history and characteristics. But it is clear that war, in all its forms, presents only negative health outcomes for the civilians and combatants directly involved, while inflicting endless financial drain on other stakeholders—from the nations doing the fighting to the humanitarian agencies tasked with cleaning up the mess.

I want us to ask: Is this what we should expect? Have thousands of years of human development, from our initial, clumsy attempts at art and language to refrigerators that can reorder our groceries, left us with war as a standard of civilization, when there is so much evidence of its futility and destructiveness? The only outcomes war guarantees are violence, oppression, and neglect of other priorities. So, what are we doing?

CHAPTER I

WAR
IS AN
EPIDEMIC

Man is stumbling blindly through a spiritual darkness while toying with the precarious secrets of life and death. The world has achieved brilliance without wisdom, power without conscience. Ours is a world of nuclear giants and ethical infants. We know more about war than we know about peace, more about killing than we know about living. This is our twentieth century's claim to distinction and to progress!

—OMAR BRADLEY,
first chairman of the Joint Chiefs of Staff of the United States (1948)

Civilization? Ha, I call it as I see it.

—OPERATION IVY, "Unity" (1989)

YEARS AFTER THE ONSET of a deadly and devastating pandemic, the idea that war in any way resembles the spread of infectious disease may seem a bit inaccurate, even hyperbolic. You can't sneeze and spread war—war isn't some contagious pathogen you can catch by touching a doorknob. We understand war as the result of choices made by people, some with good intentions and some with bad, and we attribute the trajectory of war in any given region or locality to some random mix of history, culture, economy, and bad luck that we can't easily control. We don't choose to do it; it just happens. Despite our best efforts, it's inevitable. It's human nature, right?

War is a collective form of political violence. For a long time, the field of political science studied the causes of specific wars through a historical lens; that's still how most of us learn about wars and other international affairs today. We're taught that the assassination of Archduke Franz Ferdinand of Austria was the first in a series of events that led to World War I, and we may remember that it led to the complete upheaval of not one but four empires. But the rest of it—the murder of more than nine million people, the overt racism (US president Woodrow Wilson called for the preservation of "white civilization and its domination of the planet" in 1917), the hunger and famine, the torture and sexual violence, the exploitation of Indigenous and colonized peoples, even the perpetuation of a genocide—these are learned in bits and pieces, if learned at all (Xu, 2017). To some scholars, World War I represented a sea change in how violence is perpetuated in war, as evidenced by the killing of prisoners of war and of combatants injured on the battlefield, the use of chemical weapons, and just the sheer scale of civilian deaths and internments (Jones, 2015). But most of us never learned about this purposeful application of political violence and deprivation in any meaningful way.

The violence and long-term effects of wars on people have not, historically, been treated as worthy of study in and of themselves. Early political science focused on wars between countries (interstate wars) as opposed to other forms of conflict and violence that were considered more "unconventional," like genocide, ethnic cleansing, and terrorism, which do not always occur within a neatly defined armed conflict. Violence against civilians, especially, was most often reported as an unfortunate side effect of war rather than part and parcel of a political or economic strategy. When violence against civilians was undeniable, it was treated as a practice employed during rivalries, driven by irrational hatreds, and carried out by particularly wanton or crazed actors, or as evidence of some "clash of civilizations" (Valentino, 2014).

The war that people in the Western world understand the most about is probably World War II. In school, we learn a thing or two about Mussolini and about what happened at Pearl Harbor. We're taught that Adolf Hitler and the Nazis engaged in mass extermination as part of their plan to occupy and control Europe and enact their vision of the supremacy of the Aryan race. Hitler is presented as a uniquely sinister maniac who somehow coerced an entire society, with all its complex infrastructure, to carry out his vision of extermination and supremacy, which of course was hidden from the good people of the rest of the world.

But the Nazis did not just enslave and kill Jews, Slavs, Roma, sexual minorities, and people with disabilities; they systematically dehumanized them, tortured them, and inflicted on them unimaginable acts of cruelty. The Nazis who worked at the concentration camps and carried out these acts were not unrecognizable monsters; they looked like regular people, as evidenced by the infamous photos of SS guards laughing, singing, and even decorating a Christmas tree at a concentration camp, as thousands of Jews were likely being tortured, murdered, and cremated nearby. How can "regular" people possibly justify these acts to themselves?

This is true of history's great conflicts: the violence and cruelty, the creative forms of damage to the human body, are, to some degree, part of the point. Perhaps even more uncomfortably, this level of violence is often not possible without the tacit or explicit permission and involvement of a lot of regular, everyday people. How can we explain this? How can actions that would otherwise be unjustifiable and unimaginable become very real and wholly justified by the people perpetrating them?

Are there ways to describe this phenomenon as something other than a mass delusion or even a mass sickness? Surely, you cannot solve such a sickness with a few bombs and diplomatic summits. No matter the justification, violence—acts of which are intended solely to hurt or kill—is clearly a purposeful tool of war, not an unwelcome intruder. Indeed, much of modern-day international relations is making clear that, at the right time and for the right reason, violence is always possible. We call it "saber-rattling" or "beating the drum of war," as if it were some sort of political strategy. But it's really just violence.

Our definitions of peace and conflict changed in the twentieth century for many reasons, primarily as a result of the two world wars. Many of today's international organizations were founded during this era, and multiple treaties, agreements, and guidelines on the practices of war and conflict were established. Similarly, our view of public health shifted, as our understanding of hygiene, infection, and other health factors was changing rapidly.

Aside from these advancements in science and medicine, the horrors of World War I pushed the medical community to an even more targeted understanding of the role of health in conflict and violence; and the use of amputations, ambulances, field surgery, antiseptics, and anesthesia evolved quickly. Previously, medical treatment of soldiers was nearly barbaric, and unnecessary amputations were a leading cause of death, mostly due to infections such as gangrene. Wounded soldiers were crammed into uncovered trains to be shipped to hospitals by the hundreds, with no food or water. Because the weapons of war were now so advanced, so too was the damage to bodies. The field of medicine urgently needed to keep up with this damage. In 1917, a French physician summed up this newfound calling in a talk given at a conference at a hospital in France: "Science has perfected the art of killing: Why not that of saving?" (Hampton, 2017).

When, mere decades later, World War II saw even more violent atrocities, some health professionals sought to expand the definition of health to be more holistic, to include factors like violence. For example, a 1962 paper called for the effects of violence to be considered within the purview of public health professionals (and not only that of lawyers, politicians, or the military) because it was obvious that violence significantly impedes our efforts at "extending life" and experiencing well-being (Gomez, 1962). In 1966, after decades of such advocacy by public health professionals, and a few more wars and other violent events, prevention of violence was finally recognized as a public health priority by the World Health Assembly (Krug, Mercy, Dahlberg, & Zwi, 2002). They called for a wide range of actions, such as improving both recognition of and reporting on violence, promoting public health research on violence, and pushing for greater involvement of the health sector in preventing and managing violence (WHA, 1996).

The field has grown significantly in the decades since, but there remains a pervasive view in society that the role of health professionals should be primarily reactive and clinical. Advocating for the prevention of war and other issues deemed "too political" is sometimes seen as betraying their role as neutral actors. This view is reflected in a *National Review* article from 2018: "I don't want my doctor asking me if I have guns or preaching to me about firearms policy . . . I don't want to hear my doctor pontificating about the Affordable Care Act or what our public policy should be about the opioid epidemic" (Smith, 2018). The harms inherent in our system, and the policies that might assuage them, aren't the business of health professionals, this viewpoint contends. Just keep the pills coming.

Our increased societal understanding of the social and political determinants of health, however, shows how narrow and unhealthy this viewpoint is. So, shouldn't we treat war, which is likely the most disruptive and potentially traumatic life event any person or group could possibly experience, as not just a political process but as a health catastrophe? Shouldn't we consider violence—the mechanism by which most war is waged, no matter its stated political purpose—as an urgent matter for health personnel, not just in healing wounds but in preventing them? Of course we should. And if we do so, not only will we prevent harm in areas of active war; we will also make room for transformation in societies that will deemphasize militarism and impunity and prioritize social needs and justice.

WHAT IS VIOLENCE?

Before we can understand war as a public health problem, we must understand violence. It is one of those concepts that seems so obvious, especially in the environment of war. Just look at posters for war movies: in tones of gray, green, blue, and/or brown, our hero is almost always carrying a gun, sitting at a turret, or dramatically escaping a bomb blast. "War is hell," as the infamous saying popularized by Union Army General William Tecumseh Sherman goes, and we innately know exactly what that means: it's bloody and brutal. Ugly things happen, often to people who did nothing whatsoever wrong.

International humanitarian law doesn't use the terms "war" or "civil war" but instead identifies different forms of "armed conflict," where the phrase alone insinuates the physical violence associated with conflict, war, or whatever we want to call it. Further, to be recognized by the law as an armed conflict, the groups involved need to be, not surprisingly, armed and must have some degree of organization, and their violence has to have a certain level of intensity. That means there are a lot of other forms of collective violence that do not rise to the legal definition of armed conflict, including riots, acts of terrorism, individual skirmishes, and "unrest" or "tensions" in places where the situation is potentially escalating to a precarious level.

As we'll explore in the next few chapters, there are forms of violence that don't require a weapon at all, but we cannot discount the role of weapons in perpetuating war and causing massive destruction to life and infrastructure. Indeed, the trafficking of these weapons, whether illicit or legal, is thought to be a major contributor to modern warfare. Ultimately, the direct violence so associated with conflict, from the earliest groups of humans who found something to fight over, has always been used to impose power over another group. Mao Zedong, who, as chairman of the Chinese Communist Party, presided over the deaths of tens of millions of people, made this philosophy clear: "Political power grows out of the barrel of a gun" (Li, 1995).

While the concept of violence seems straightforward, the typology is actually quite complex. *The World Report on Violence and Health*, published by the World Health Organization (WHO) after the World Health Assembly in 1996, defines violence as "the intentional use of physical force or power, threatened or actual, against oneself, another person, or against a group or community, that either results in or has a high likelihood of resulting in injury, death, psychological harm, maldevelopment or deprivation." This offers a multilayered view of violence involving a host of different actors, victims, and outcomes. In this definition, there are three categories of violence, depending on the actor: collective, interpersonal, and self-directed. Then there is the nature of the violence itself: physical, sexual, psychological, or deprivation/neglect (Rutherford, Zwi, Grove, & Butchart, 2007). These forms of violence often intersect and overlap, as will become clear in the chapters that follow.

The nature of the actor perpetrating the violence offers another cross-section through which to view violence, one that has become increasingly important in the public health literature. Violence, in fact, requires an actor. Despite a potentially high death toll and significant harm to infrastructure, we would not consider an earthquake or tsunami to be an act of violence. Yet violence can be present through other mechanisms, ones we might currently regard as random or inevitable. As Johan Galtung, a prominent Norwegian peace researcher, noted, "If a person died from tuberculosis in the eighteenth century it would be hard to conceive of this as violence since it might have been quite unavoidable, but if he dies from it today, despite all the medical resources in the world, then violence is present." As such, Galtung further clarifies two additional forms of violence: direct, and indirect (or structural) (Galtung, 1969).

Direct violence is an academic term, but one of the few whose meaning is clear upon a first reading. It is exactly as it sounds—direct. There is an actor (or actors) directly harming a victim (or victims). This is what is popularly considered "real" violence: not just shooting and bombing, but rape, torture, and domestic abuse.

Indirect violence, on the other hand, cannot often be traced back to an individual actor directly harming another. In this form of violence, the harm is baked into structures in the form of power imbalances, inequities, and deprivation. Unlike with direct violence, witnesses and even victims may not perceive indirect violence at all, or may even deem these forms of structural violence as acceptable. Though not a health scholar, Galtung differentiates these inequities clearly through health-related examples: "In a society where life expectancy is twice as high in the upper as in the lower classes, violence is exercised even if there are no concrete actors one can point to directly attacking others, as when one person kills another" (Galtung, 1969). It is through these typologies that, in the coming chapters, we will advance our discussion of violence as a tool of war and a threat to public health.

VIOLENCE, WAR, AND PUBLIC HEALTH

The World Health Assembly in 1996 helped solidify an emerging wave of research and practice on violence and health. This meant that, rather than studying war only in terms of politics and history, we now saw wider adoption of public health frameworks and practices in areas of violence. In 1997, two physicians, Barry Levy and Victor Sidel (a cofounder, in 1961, of Physicians for Social Responsibility), edited the first major book on the relationship between war and public health. The authors, a group of physicians and public health scholars, contributed dozens of chapters on a host of health considerations relating to war, including mental health, the environment, the effects of weapons, and the unique needs of children, women, detainees, and the displaced. Importantly, they identified the responsibility of public health professionals to act as credible voices in the calls against violence and armed conflict, not only because of the effect of violence on human life but also because societies that narrowly define security as a well-stocked and well-trained military tend to divert attention and resources from other basic human needs. This book was groundbreaking in the field of public health, and the authors became well known for their writings on the health consequences of war and other societal ills, like climate change and social injustice. Their works were among the first to motivate many scholars, myself included, to understand war as a public health problem that, like any disease or ailment, can be prevented.

Other physicians and public health officials took the lead in making the practical connections between violence and health. Dr. Gary Slutkin, an epidemiologist, professor, and advisor to the World Health Organization, treated epidemics in refugee camps early in his career. Over time, he began to recognize violence, specifically gun violence, as akin to an infectious disease, even an epidemic. He founded Cure Violence, an organization that uses a disease control model to prevent community violence, in 2000. In 2009, the American Public Health Association, the oldest and largest organization of public health professionals in the world, adopted a resolution naming war as a public health problem. Two years later, to address the prevention of armed conflict and militarism, they formed the Public Health Working Group on Primary Prevention of War, which I joined early in my academic career. These are just some of the examples of the emergence of this field in recent decades. Yet, while the research base is growing, the ideas, policies, and warnings of these experts and groups have largely gone unheeded.

Because public health involves both clinical and social factors, there are many models for understanding health promotion, action, and impact. In terms of prevention, however, the typical approach adopts a model with three levels: primary, secondary, and tertiary prevention (CDC, 2017). Most health systems today, including in the conflict-affected context, emphasize tertiary prevention, which means managing health outcomes only after a diagnosis or incident. This level of prevention is costly and difficult to apply equitably, especially in events of mass casualties. Secondary prevention, on the other hand, includes enhanced screening processes to identify and treat disease as early as possible. Primary prevention requires intervention before the health problem occurs at all. This approach demands collective efforts, all rooted in evidence and equity, from individuals, groups, and policymakers alike.

Looking at smoking, for example, primary prevention might include banning smoking in certain areas, limiting nicotine advertising, and increasing education on smoking hazards. Secondary prevention could focus on enhanced screening for smokers and the promotion of smoking cessation or nicotine replacement therapies; while tertiary prevention could entail pharmaceutical or surgical interventions to manage lung cancer.

This model has been applied to many forms of violence, including sexual violence, child maltreatment, intimate partner violence, gun violence, and crime. Not surprisingly, then, it has been applied to the context of political violence and armed conflict. A 2010 article presented a multitiered approach to intervention in conflict, considering the massive number of stakeholders at any given level (De Jong, 2010). In this case, tertiary prevention—the equivalent of surgery in the lung cancer model—involves preventing already occurring wars from becoming long-lasting, and includes reconstruction and rehabilitation efforts. Many billions of dollars have been invested at this level, mimicking our reactive health systems.

At the secondary level, we might emphasize early crisis intervention and activating mechanisms that enforce accountability at the United Nations and other bodies. Lastly, primary prevention, in this context, would focus on preventing conflicts from happening in the first place. This includes tackling some of the most deeply rooted societal ills: inequalities, lack of education, poverty, rural underdevelopment, and the stifling of a free press, to cite just a few examples.

The primary level may be the most significant, but it is also the hardest to envision. How is it possible to prevent all potential conflicts from occurring in a world with billions of people? The real answer to this question is that, of course, we cannot. But that being so has led us to undervalue the many interventions that could both significantly reduce outbreaks of war and improve population health and well-being. War is treated as inevitable in ways we treat almost nothing else. It is more possible today to fathom taking a leisure trip to the moon than it is to imagine a world with little to no war, or even a world in which global powers hold each other accountable to the same standard when transgressions occur.

Although crafting a world with no political, social, or economic frictions may be impossible, by accepting war as an inevitability, we let ourselves off the hook for preventing it, punishing those who perpetrate it, and meaningfully serving those affected by it. Maybe we can't prevent all wars. We cannot prevent all diseases or injuries either, no matter our individual wealth and comforts. But while it is possible for an individual who has never smoked to get lung cancer, or for a driver wearing a seat belt to be killed in a car accident, we still engage in massive public health and safety campaigns to prevent smoking and increase the use of seat belts. Why aren't we doing the same with war?

Some scholars argue that in limiting our understanding of violence to that of a "disease," we actually miss the nuance of how violence manifests in societies (Williams & Donnelly, 2014). But if we can begin to understand violence, including political violence, as a multifaceted phenomenon with many potential areas for intervention and prevention—as we only recently have with other health-related issues—we can expand our thinking about what can be done to prevent it. In understanding war as a public health problem, other analogues to the disease model become possible, including the perception that violence is contagious.

We often underestimate the spread of violence. It is not random. Further, when violence goes unchecked, or is seemingly permitted or even encouraged by powerful entities, it becomes normalized. This changes how a society views violence. When citizens feel ignored, or feel as though they don't have access to traditional methods of justice, they are more likely to turn to violence. They may even come to view victims of violence as deserving of it, or as more likely to be perpetrators than victims (Kleinfeld & Barham, 2018).

In 2012, the US Institute of Medicine held the Forum on Global Violence Prevention (2013) to explore evidence-based epidemiological approaches as applied to violence. They assessed the transmission of violence, using examples of community riots and mass killings like those in Rwanda. They also looked at the evidence of how early exposure to violence can increase the likelihood of perpetuating violence as an adult, and considered the increased risk of suicide after exposure to a suicide in a peer group or in media reports. They considered physiological and social processes that can increase risk of individual or group violence. It is a highly referenced and comprehensive report that concludes that violence is analogous to a contagious disease in many ways, while acknowledging that the status quo does not fully appreciate this reality.

WAR IS AN EPIDEMIC

I had the idea for this book in 2018; like most acts of writing, it took a little time before it was well-developed enough to come to fruition. My proposal was accepted in early 2020, and I had fantastical plans to travel to conflict-affected settings to conduct interviews and make observations in hospitals dealing with victims of political violence. Then, a few weeks after I had signed my contract, global travel was shut down. The mysterious virus that we had heard hints about for months was no longer mysterious. It was, in fact, a pandemic, according to the World Health Organization. Schools were closed; the skies were clear of airplanes. A trip to the grocery store, if one was fortunate enough to still have resources to buy food, became an event to prepare for, with masks and gloves and hand sanitizer. Suddenly, everyone knew what a pandemic was. The Merriam-Webster Word of 2020 was "pandemic." Dictionary.com chose the word "unprecedented." Both appropriate, in my view.

How then, to make the argument that war, and not the pandemic (ongoing as I write this), is the greatest threat to public health? Indeed, how to compare war to a pandemic at all? Instead of the pandemic undermining my argument, however, I continued to find evidence that armed conflict and political violence are more detrimental to human life—and even more similar to a disease—than I had originally proposed. Further, it was obvious that political tension, conflict, and nationalism had made us even more vulnerable to the pandemic. What might have happened, had China been more forthcoming about the mysterious virus they had been tracking in late 2019? Would we have had a Delta wave, if vaccines had been distributed equitably from the beginning? Would vaccine hesitancy have been lower if people had trusted their governments more? Who is ultimately responsible for the health of the millions of people living in war or under siege, or the millions more who are displaced and stateless?

The COVID-19 pandemic has forced many to learn a public health vocabulary that we might have rather left as esoteric. One of these terms is "endemic," which is the amount of disease that is standard in a community, also known as the baseline level. Disease is present, but predictable. Malaria, for example, is considered endemic in certain parts of Africa, and some sexually transmitted infections are considered endemic in parts of the world. Some have classified violence against women and girls as endemic (*The Lancet*, 2021). Endemic violence is also cited as a primary challenge to many countries' broader health goals (Roberts, 2018).

An epidemic, on the other hand, occurs when the number of cases exceeds what is normal. This can have many causes, including an increase in amount of the agent, the introduction of the agent into a new setting, or other factors that increase population exposure to the agent (CDC,

2012). While "epidemic" typically refers to infections that spread between people, not all epidemics do so, such as past outbreaks of Lyme disease, the West Nile virus, or the Zika virus, all of which are transmitted by insects. We've also referred to obesity, drug overdoses, and gun violence as epidemics, and they certainly are not spread through pathogens. In 2020, the president of the American Psychological Association even argued that "We are living in a racism pandemic." Yet we haven't applied this framing to war, seemingly tolerating bouts of war, and the militarization they foster, as endemic—predictable and, in many ways, acceptable—even with evidence that war may be contagious both within and between states (Lane, 2016).

In fact, evidence shows that, when one or more states are at war, opportunities and willingness to engage in war increase among other states, depending on borders, alliances, or other political factors. This has long been referred to as the "diffusion" of war (Siverson & Starr, 1990). How else to explain the aftermath of 9/11, when terrorist acts against the United States, committed by men primarily from Saudi Arabia, led to wars in Afghanistan and Iraq and resulted in the United States and countries like France and the United Kingdom bombing countries throughout the Middle East and Africa for two decades?

Like many mechanisms of contagion, there are multiple factors that may lead to diffusion of war. These include interstate ethnic linkages, even among states that are not geographically close (Buhaug & Gleditsch, 2008). And rather than proposing that this diffusion is accidental or circumstantial, some research suggests that often, when interstate wars spill across borders, it's no accident. Governments use civil wars to engage in proxy battles with neighboring states, and "can use transnationalized conflicts to strengthen their hold on the state and to gain regional superiority. The spreading of violence across borders is thus calculated and controlled" (De Maio, 2010). Neighboring states may be further destabilized by refugee flows, especially when refugee populations are marginalized and oppressed, as many are by host countries (Lischer, 2017).

Further, the spread of the weapons of war has an almost infectious pathway, where the powerful military states are in a race to acquire the same weapons as each other and produce even more threatening ones.

The new arms race is in the realm of hypersonic weapons, where China and Russia have entered the arena of outer space; likewise, the US Department of Defense is investing $1 billion per year, in addition to launching a new satellite network meant to track these weapons, which are otherwise impossible to shoot down (Stone, 2020). What might be next?

This introduces the other intersection between war and health. Health, as defined by the World Health Organization, is "a state of complete physical, mental and social well-being and not merely the absence of disease or infirmity" (1946). While having the top military budget in the world by far, the United States performs among the worst in multiple health indicators compared to other wealthy countries, despite a high health care price tag. The United States has the lowest life expectancy among the 36 OECD—high-income—countries. The United States is also the only highly developed country without universal health coverage, and has the highest suicide rates, the highest chronic disease burden, and the highest proportion of avoidable deaths (Tikkanen & Abrams, 2020).

The United States also has the top homicide rate among high-income countries, and a gun violence rate that is 25 times greater than those of its counterparts (Grinshteyn & Hemenway, 2016). Infant and maternal mortality is also the highest among peer nations (The Lancet Child & Adolescent Health, 2021), and the number of homeless children in the United States is at historic highs (NCHE, 2020).

With a string of largely unsuccessful and devastatingly costly (in lives as well as funds) wars in recent decades, the prioritizing of militarization and war at the expense of social goods has done arguably little to protect the American people. Yet this creeping militarization is only possible because of successful attempts to convince us that massive military budgets, intrusions of personal privacy and surveillance, and even the militarization of domestic police forces is really what secures us (Carpenter, 2016) and not access to health services, food, and housing.

The massive military budget of the United States (approximately $800 billion in just 2021 [World Bank, 2023]) and its comparatively poor health performance make it an easy target in such discussions, but the side effects of violence, and the militarization it necessitates, are even clearer when considered on the global scale. The Institute for Economics & Peace, which publishes the Global Peace Index and the Global Terrorism Index, estimates that global violence costs more than $14 trillion per year, equivalent to 11.6% of the world's economic activity. More than just war, this includes the cost of incarceration, crime, suicide, and other forms of violence. Armed conflict, by their calculation, costs $448 billion—only about 3% of the annual total. Homicide was less than 7%.

So where is all the money going? A full 43% of the cost is military expenditure, coming in at $6.4 trillion (IEP, 2021). Not only are violence and war akin to an epidemic in their incidence, but our investment in them prevents us from tackling the real threats to our health and well-being.

REFERENCES

American Psychological Association (APA). (2020). *"We are living in a racism pandemic,"* says APA president. https://www.apa.org/news/press/releases/2020/05/racism-pandemic.

Buhaug, H., & Gleditsch, K. S. (2008). Contagion or confusion? Why conflicts cluster in space. *International Studies Quarterly, 52*(2), 215–233. http://www.jstor.org/stable/29734233.

Centers for Disease Control and Prevention (CDC). (2012). *Section 11: epidemic disease occurrence.* https://www.cdc.gov/csels/dsepd/ss1978/lesson1/section11.html.

Centers for Disease Control and Prevention (CDC). (2017). *Picture of America: prevention.* https://www.cdc.gov/pictureofamerica/pdfs/Picture_of_America_Prevention.pdf.

De Jong, J. (2010). A public health framework to translate risk factors related to political violence and war into multi-level preventive interventions. *Social Science & Medicine, 70*(1), 71–79.

De Maio, J. (2010). Is war contagious? The transnationalization of conflict in Darfur. *African Studies Quarterly, 11*(4), 25–44.

Forum on Global Violence Prevention; Board on Global Health; Institute of Medicine; National Research Council. (2013). Violence is a contagious disease. In *Contagion of violence: workshop summary.* Washington, DC: National Academies Press.

Galtung, J. (1969). Violence, peace, and peace research. *Journal of Peace Research, 6*(3), 167–191.

Gomez, A. (1962). Violence requires epidemiological studies. *Tribuna Medica, 2,* 1–12.

Grinshteyn, E., & Hemenway, D. (2016). Violent death rates: the US compared with other high-income OECD countries, 2010. *The American Journal of Medicine*, *129*(3), 266–273. https://doi.org/10.1016/j.amjmed.2015.10.025.

Hampton, E. (2017, February 24). How World War I revolutionized medicine. *The Atlantic*. https://www.theatlantic.com/health/archive/2017/02/world-war-i-medicine/517656/.

Institute for Economics & Peace (IEP). (2021). *Global peace index 2021*. https://www.visionofhumanity.org/wp-content/uploads/2021/06/GPI-2021-web-1.pdf.

Jones, H. (2015). Violent transgression and the First World War. *Studies: An Irish Quarterly*, *104*(414), 124–143.

Kleinfeld, R., & Barham, E. (2018). Complicit states and the governing strategy of privilege violence: when weakness is not the problem. *Annual Review of Political Science*, *21*, 215–238.

Krug, E., Mercy, J., Dahlberg, L., & Zwi, A. (2002). The world report on violence and health. *The Lancet*, *360*(9339), 1083–1088.

The Lancet Child & Adolescent Health. (2021a). Endemic violence against women and girls. *The Lancet*, *5*(5), P309.

The Lancet Child & Adolescent Health. (2021b). Infant and maternal mortality in the USA. *The Lancet*, *5*(1), P1. https://doi.org/10.1016/S2352-4642(20)30369-2.

Lane, M. (2016). The intrastate contagion of ethnic civil war. *The Journal of Politics*, *78*(2), 396–410.

Li, Gucheng. (Ed.). (1995). *A Glossary of Political Terms of the People's Republic of China*. Hong Kong: The Chinese University Press.

Lischer, S. (2017). The global refugee crisis: regional destabilization & humanitarian protection. *Dædalus*. *146*(4), 85–97.

National Center for Homeless Education (NCHE). (2020). *Federal data summary: school years 2015–16 through 2017–18*. https://nche.ed.gov/wp-content/uploads/2020/01/Federal-Data-Summary-SY-15.16-to-17.18-Published-1.30.2020.pdf.

Roberts, L. F. (2018). When violence becomes endemic. *International Journal of Public Health*, *63*(Suppl 1), 3–5. https://doi.org/10.1007/s00038-017-1001-6.

Rutherford, A., Zwi, A. B., Grove, N. J., & Butchart, A. (2007). Violence: a glossary. *Journal of Epidemiology and Community Health*, *61*(8), 676–680. https://doi.org/10.1136/jech.2005.043711.

Siverson, R. M., & Starr, H. (1990). Opportunity, willingness, and the diffusion of war. *The American Political Science Review*, *84*(1), 47–67. https://doi.org/10.2307/1963629.

Smith, W. (2018, October 22). Physicians should prescribe pills, not politics. *The National Review.* https://www.nationalreview.com/corner/physicians-prescibe-pills-not-politics/.

Stewart, F. (2002). Root causes of violent conflict in developing countries. *BMJ*, 324(7333), 342–345.

Stone, R. (2020, January 8). "National pride is at stake." Russia, China, United States race to build hypersonic weapons. *Science.* https://www.science.org/content/article/national-pride-stake-russia-china-united-states-race-build-hypersonic-weapons.

Tikkanen, R., & Abrams, M. (2020, January 30). *U.S. health care from a global perspective, 2019: higher spending, worse outcomes?* Commonwealth Fund. https://www.commonwealthfund.org/publications/issue-briefs/2020/jan/us-health-care-global-perspective-2019.

Valentino, B. (2014). Why we kill: the political science of political violence against civilians. *Annual Review of Political Science, 17,* 89–103. https://doi.org/10.1146/annurev-polisci-082112-141937.

Williams, D., & Donnelly, P. (2014). Is violence a disease? Situating violence prevention in public health policy and practice. *Public Health, 128*(11), 960–967.

World Bank. (2023). Military expenditure (current USD)—United States. https://data.worldbank.org/indicator/MS.MIL.XPND.CD?locations=US.

World Health Assembly (WHA). (1996). *WHA49.25 Prevention of violence: a public health priority.* https://apps.who.int/iris/handle/10665/179463.

World Health Organization (WHO). (1946). *WHO Constitution.* https://www.who.int/about/governance/constitution.

Xu, Guoqi. (2017). *Asia and the Great War.* Oxford: Oxford University Press.

CHAPTER 2

HEALTH IS POLITICAL

I wish those people who write so glibly about this being a holy War, and the orators who talk so much about going on no matter how long the War lasts and what it may mean, could see a case—to say nothing of 10 cases—of mustard gas in its early stages—could see the poor things burnt and blistered all over with great mustard-colored suppurating blisters, with blind eyes—sometimes temporally, sometimes permanently—all sticky and stuck together, and always fighting for breath, with voices a mere whisper, saying that their throats are closing and they know they will choke.

—VERA BRITTAIN, nurse during World War I (1933)

War, I despise
'Cause it means destruction of innocent lives
War means tears to thousands of mothers' eyes
When their sons go off to fight
And lose their lives.

—EDWIN STARR, "War" (1970)

LESS THAN FOUR DECADES AGO, two of the world's biggest powers, the United States and the Soviet Union, seemed to be on a path to a war. Not *only* war, but catastrophic nuclear war that could decimate entire population centers, as the United States itself had perpetrated in Nagasaki and Hiroshima in 1945. In those incidents, aside from the tens of thousands of Japanese civilians killed in the immediate blast, thousands died in the months afterward due to injuries or complications from acute radiation syndrome. In the 50 years after the bombings, higher-than-normal rates of cancers for those who survived the attack claimed hundreds more lives. Americans were worried about suffering a similar fate at the hands of the Soviet Union, leading to duck-and-cover drills in schools and commercially sold personal fallout shelters for homes. While it is evident today that these measures would likely have done little to protect one's safety in the event of a direct nuclear attack, the sentiment was clear: people were terrified of being killed or injured in an attack by a foreign adversary.

In the early 1980s, a group of six physicians (three each from the United States and the Soviet Union) came together in the mutual under-standing that their "common interest in survival was more powerful than the ideological divides between them" (IPPNW, 2017). To advocate this message, they formed an organization that was the first of its kind: International Physicians for the Prevention of Nuclear War (IPPNW). These doctors worked together to conduct medical studies based on data from the bombing sites in Hiroshima and Nagasaki. This followed a special is-sue of the famed *New England Journal of Medicine* written by several early members of IPPNW in 1962, which had a very clear answer to any suggestion that this work was not a physician's place. Why should doc-tors care about this seemingly political stuff? According to these physi-cians, "No single group is as deeply involved in and committed to the sur-vival of mankind. No group is as accustomed to the labor of applying the practical solutions to life-threatening difficulties" (Nathan, Geiger, Sidel, & Lown, 1962). Based on the research done by these doctors, they came to a straightforward conclusion: in the event of a nuclear war, there was no medical response, no cure, no treatment.

They took a very quantitative, evidence-based approach. This was not a case of some doctors yelling from a soapbox but rather a frank con-sideration of the factors physicians would have to contend with in the event of a thermonuclear attack: "How many persons will be killed out-right? How many will be fatally injured? How many will be injured, but survive? Similarly, how many physicians will be killed or injured? Will any necessary medical supplies . . . be left? And where will physicians, patients, beds and supplies be in relation to one another?" (Sidel, Geiger, & Lown, 1962). In the words of former New Zealand Prime Minister David Lange, "IPPNW made medical reality a part of political reality" (IPPNW, n.d.).

IPPNW spent its first few years on growing its network, which included its US affiliate, Physicians for Social Responsibility (PSR), educating the public, health practitioners, and politicians about the medical consequences of nuclear war. Only four years after its inception, IPPNW won the UNESCO Peace Education Prize; and a year later, in 1985, the group won the Nobel Peace Prize for their advocacy and research. Since then, they have released many groundbreaking reports and have expanded their mandate to prevent military conflicts of any kind and to explore the relationships between peace and health (Nobel Peace Summit, 2019). Today, they have affiliates around the world, from Argentina to Zambia, composed of medical professionals who explicitly denounce political policies that could lead to human catastrophes.

The organization Physicians for Human Rights (PHR) was founded in 1986 by doctors who had witnessed atrocities and human rights violations in Chile, Vietnam, apartheid South Africa, and Argentina. PHR has an approach that is similar to that of IPPNW: document, advocate, and empower. On the other hand, organizations like Médecins Sans Frontières (MSF, founded in 1971 and known in English as Doctors without Borders) and the International Medical Corps (IMC, founded in 1984) emphasize neutrality and impartiality, and both of these consider their priorities to be medical-first. By focusing on delivering care at the expense of all other considerations, these organizations attest that they can gain access to the most vulnerable populations and save more lives by remaining relief organizations, as opposed to spilling into human rights or justice activism. However, these organizations do try to raise awareness of humanitarian crises, which includes conducting research on significant and often overlooked humanitarian issues.

In practice, to maintain their access, these organizations have sometimes gone so far as to pay armed militias for permission to work in territories they hold or even to apologize to a government for including their country (i.e., Yemen) in a "Top Ten Humanitarian Crises" list. Despite how this might sound from an outsider's perspective, the Yemeni government did immediately lift the sanctions they'd imposed on MSF, allowing MSF to fulfill their number-one goal: reaching patients (Magone, Neuman, & Weissman, 2012). A stance built on zero engagement with antagonists might, potentially, have been persuasive in some unknown long term; but, in the immediate present, there were people suffering who needed aid. When accepting the 1999 Nobel Peace Prize on behalf of the organization, then-MSF President Dr. James Orbinski said, "The humanitarian act is the most apolitical of all acts, but if its actions and its morality are taken seriously, it has the most profound of political implications."

So, what's the right answer? Attend to needy and vulnerable patients, even if that means, at times, appeasing authoritarian and repressive regimes? Or advocate against the actors and policies that have led these populations to their vulnerable state, even if that means losing access to them in the meantime? This same dilemma—just how political should health care be?—plays out in public health deliberations in all contexts. Scholars, practitioners, and advocates who might agree with the MSF and IMC approach argue that a "harm reduction" strategy is needed: work to save lives now. In other words, it's someone else's job to fix the big stuff. Their counterparts in PHR (who themselves shared in the 1997 Nobel Peace Prize) and PSR see their role as not just to conduct research or expose human rights violations, but to hold perpetrators accountable and end impunity. These are inherently political, and sometimes controversial, acts.

Of course, in terms of these organizations and the many others like them, there is no real tension in their coexistence. Each plays a role in the ecosystem of humanitarian response, and each has its own critics and champions. Fundamental to the entire humanitarian response sector—which in 2018 required a quarter of a trillion dollars just to meet baseline needs—is the fact that the majority (up to 80%) of the world's humanitarian needs are a direct consequence of conflict. Ending, or at least reducing, conflicts in the world would save countless lives and money, and would allow for long-term development, instead of constant emergency spending.

Importantly, however, shifting global attention away from national security (e.g., the focus on military dominance) and toward human security (food, shelter, health, and other aspects of a decent and dignified life) might provide the political bandwidth to generate solutions for emerging global challenges, such as climate change, aging populations, and automation. Overcoming these looming concerns will require, at a minimum, global collective action on a scale we have never seen.

All this sounds strikingly obvious. And together, the world bodies, many of which were built in the wreckage of the Second World War (e.g., the United Nations, World Health Organization, World Bank, International Monetary Fund) rhetorically understand this. They've all issued reports, statements, case studies, and press releases about how detrimental war is to human life and development at all stages. And yet, year after year, states make their real priorities known by inflating military budgets while reducing funding for humanitarian causes and social services, which they see as ancillary. While this trend is global, the United States is a prime example. A recent study found that since 2001, the United States has spent at least $6.4 trillion on wars in Afghanistan, Iraq, Syria, and Pakistan. The "war on terror" justification has also been used for other expensive operations, not only the search for the supposed weapons of mass destruction we were supposed to find in Iraq, but in countries like the Philippines (Crawford, 2019).

And although the United States is by far the largest single contributor to humanitarian aid in the world, in 2019 the United States cut humanitarian spending by 6%, despite an all-time high in the number of people requiring humanitarian interventions (Development Initiatives, 2019). For its own people, the United States expends only 18.7% of the GDP on social spending—less than the mean for developed countries, which is 20.1% (OECD, 2019). Meanwhile, the US Census Bureau reports that 8.5% of Americans had no health insurance in 2018, a decline from those covered in 2017—including an additional 425,000 uninsured children—due to a reduction in public coverage (Berchick & Mykyta, 2019). While maternal mortality is declining in much of the world, it is actually increasing in the United States, where it is already the highest among high-income countries (Global Burden of Disease, 2016). The trillions of dollars earmarked for wars that never seem to end could make a significant difference, if only those dollars could be allocated to other sectors.

The cruel reality of our modern, sophisticated times is that, instead of deeming the practice of war to be outdated, we have instead modernized how we *do* war: with drones, "surgical strikes," even "nonlethal weapons" like sponge-tipped bullets and tear gas. We have entire industries whose only goal is to make conflict sleeker, shinier, and less lethal to those states that can afford these weapons, while of course making it much more dangerous for their adversaries. Instead of merely bombing population centers—still quite popular among bad actors with access to an air force—nation-states and armed groups have mastered other forms of direct and structural violence, like sieges; extrajudicial assassinations; disrupted food, water, and sanitation systems; and the eradication or propagandization of education.

To respond to the threats of potential nuclear winter or biological warfare, the world's billionaires aren't putting their resources into peace or development promotion policies—they're building bunkers in New Zealand, and custom-fitting Gulfstream jets to aid in their quick escape (Carville, 2018). Yet the "peace industry," whose key goals are to prevent costly wars, promote the use of diplomatic and political levers, and maintain human dignity and well-being, consists mostly of a fragmented sector of academics, a few scholarly and advocacy organizations, the aforementioned humanitarian and relief industries, and the occasional politician who argues for pacifism and the end of the military-industrial complex. People and groups, in other words, who are often seen as unrealistic hippies or outliers on the political fringe. The revived bunker industry, I'm sure, agrees.

So are we just to accept that war—the number-one driver of humanitarian needs; the impetus behind the forced migration of millions of people; the arena in which some of the world's biggest companies make billions of dollars; and the sector that diverts nations' spending from health, education, and infrastructure to military and defense budgets—is the standard? War has become an acceptable norm, treated as "background noise," contends Dr. Amy Hagopian from the University of Washington. She argues that, instead of treating war as a preventable public health issue, like tobacco and car accidents, the health sector primarily sees its role in war or conflict as one of medical response.

This assumption then plays out in the dearth of peer-reviewed journals, grants, college departments and classes, and conferences that focus on war as a public health problem (Hagopian, 2017). This further devalues the field as an area of pursuit for academics and practitioners, which in turn leads to a vacuum of health-focused policy, deprioritizing solutions for conflict that are outside of the "medical-first" approach.

Popular culture perpetuates this bias, further reinforcing the idea that, while things aren't perfect, they are better than at any other point in mankind's history—leading to the assumption that we don't have to take any extraordinary steps for change. In 2011, psychologist Steven Pinker published the book *The Better Angels of Our Nature: Why Violence Has Declined*. Perhaps you've heard his argument, which is straightforward: based on statistics gauging worldwide battle deaths per 100,000 people, our current period is one of the most peaceful in human history. Yes, there is still war, but it only seems more visible today because of the incentives of mass media and other dynamics. Pinker points to several "civilizing" trends, such as increases in women's empowerment and the power of the state, as well as changes in the trajectory of mankind from violent tribes who committed human sacrifice to nation-states who embrace democracy (sometimes).

Pinker's book was widely publicized around the time that we started to witness such events as the deterioration in Syria that led to the ongoing civil war; the death of Gaddafi and a new period of destabilization for Libya; violence in South Sudan that has since been referred to as a genocide; and an increase in violence in Iraq that ushered in the Islamic State of Iraq and Syria (ISIS), among many other conflicts. Pinker's position drew critique from other academics, resulting in several counter-articles published in the wake of his book. In 2015, for example, Cirillo and Taleb argued that the current "long peace" Pinker claims we're experiencing is really just a statistical sampling error that portends no information about the future; while Falk and Hildebolt (2017) argue that people in the smaller societies of the past were not more violent, but just had a higher likelihood of being killed in conflict because there were fewer people in general. They believe that innovations in weaponry and military strategy have actually made it easier to kill in modern warfare. Meanwhile, Oka et al. (2017) found that war-related casualties are better described by population scaling (i.e., how large is the group at war) and related factors, like logistical considerations and available technology. They also caution against using the minimally available information about historical violence to make comparisons or propose trends with the much more well-documented violence of today.

Ultimately, the data tells us that Pinker is likely correct that fewer people overall are dying as a result of active conflict than in the twentieth century. However, the actual number of armed conflicts is steadily increasing, with approximately 55 active conflicts across dozens of countries in 2022. As one report on these phenomena summarized, "fewer people are killed in fewer wars, but there are more low-level conflicts that potentially can spiral out of control" (Strand, Rustad, Urdal, & Nygard, 2019). This makes it hard to truly feel any sense of "long peace," especially as so many more states seem poised to tip into fragility or even armed conflict. While overall global mortality as a result of war has technically declined, war has become increasingly concentrated in low- and middle-income countries in the Middle East and Africa, home to 26 of the 37 states identified as fragile or conflict-affected.

There are dozens of languages spoken, religions practiced, and ethnicities present throughout the different states of the Middle East and Africa, though these states are often lumped together as a singular region. What does connect them is a deep, and quite recent, history of colonialism. Studies show that colonialism is linked to ethnic conflicts in Africa (Blanton, Mason, & Athow, 2001) and the Middle East (Del Sarto, 2017), and colonized states that historically depended on labor exploitation now report between 15% and 30% lower gross domestic product (GDP) per capita than other states (Bruhn & Gallego, 2012).

Colonialism served to entrench massive inequalities in these societies, bolstered by lower public investment (Engerman & Sokoloff, 2005), and colonizers brought their own principles of Western health systems—primarily for their own benefit and to promote their own interests—overriding local culture and customs, which widened health disparities between themselves and indigenous populations (Lasker, 1977). Generally, a history of colonialism has negative impacts on the health of the populations in low-income countries, in part due to generational malnutrition (Turshen, 1977); insidiously, though, the process of colonization weakens the state to the point that populations begin to depend on their colonizers for medical services, in turn legitimizing colonial control (Manderson, 1987). Thus, as theorist Frantz Fanon (born in the French colony of Martinique) argues in his pivotal work *The Wretched of the Earth*, "The colonized, underdeveloped man is today a political creature in the most global sense of the term" (p. 40). It follows that factors affecting these people's everyday lives, including quite literally their mortality, are inherently political, as well.

WHAT IS A FRAGILE OR CONFLICT-AFFECTED STATE?

Although they seem like straightforward concepts, war, conflict, and fragility in a country can be complex to define. Even within the peace and conflict literature, there are many definitions of war, including types of war (cold/hot war, civil or international war, proxy war, preventive war, and so on) and forms of warfare (biological, economic, cyber, guerrilla, etc.). There are just as many definitions for peace, which most scholars agree is not simply the absence of war. Although shows of physical force and coercion are certainly factors in almost all wars, war is not limited to brute violence. War is ultimately a political process, undertaken when two or more actors aim to settle a dispute or otherwise remedy some ills, usually with the intent to harm the other party out of malice, to exert pressure, or some combination of both. Different forms of violence are used to carry out these goals. But as military strategist Bernard Brodie, one of the architects of American postures of nuclear deterrence, described, "Although war represents human violence in its most intensive form, it is not simply human violence" (1973).

The term "fragile states" has been widely used in the 2000s by major global organizations, like the World Health Organization, the World Bank, and the Organisation for Economic Co-operation and Development (OECD). The OECD defines fragile states as those that "suffer

TABLE I.

Fragile and Conflict-Affected States, 2023 (by WHO region)

AFRO (17)	EMRO (9)	WPRO (5)	AMRO (2)	EURO (2)	SEARO (2)
Burundi	Afghanistan	Marshall Islands	Haiti	Kosovo[†]	Myanmar
Burkina Faso	Iraq	Micronesia, Federated States	Venezuela	Ukraine	Timor-Leste
Cameroon	Lebanon				
Central African Republic	Libya	Papua New Guinea			
Chad	Occupied Palestinian Territory[*]	Solomon Islands			
Comoros	Somalia	Tuvalu			
Congo, Democratic Republic	Sudan				
Congo, Republic	Syrian Arab Republic				
Eritrea	Yemen				
Ethiopia					
Guinea-Bissau					
Mali					
Mozambique					
Niger					
Nigeria					
South Sudan					
Zimbabwe					

Note: AFRO = African Region; AMRO = Americas Region; EMRO = Eastern Mediterranean Region; EURO = European Region; SEARO = South-East Asian Region; WPRO = Western Pacific Region
* Referred to as "West Bank and Gaza" by the World Bank
† Not formally recognized by WHO

deficits in governance, reflecting the internal dynamics of a society, or exogenous factors such as natural disasters and regional conflict," where governments are unable or unwilling "to perform key state functions for the benefit of all" (2008). Fragile states do not have to feature active conflict, although state fragility often leads to, or is the result of, conflict. See table 1 for a regional breakdown of fragile and conflict-affected states.

The relationship between fragility and conflict seems clear. So, what is conflict then? Here, the definitions are a bit more precise, because the type of conflict opens the door to international humanitarian law, which recognizes two types: international armed conflict and non-international armed conflict. International armed conflict is conflict between two nations, like the war between North Korea and South Korea in the 1950s, or between Russia and Ukraine more recently. We see fewer of these today, and that's no accident. The international order that we know—the United Nations, NATO, and the like, which grew out of the post–World War II period—with all its flaws and shortcomings, exists primarily to prevent these catastrophic wars.

Non-international armed conflict, on the other hand, is defined as extended armed confrontation between governmental armed forces and the forces of one or more organized armed groups (like the civil war in Syria, with the Syrian government fighting various Syrian armed groups on Syrian territory), or conflict between two or more non-state actors on a state's territory. This typology can be very complicated. For example, the war in Afghanistan, despite involving many global actors, including the United States, was widely classified as a non-international armed conflict, because the war was technically between the Afghan government (supported by foreign militaries) and armed groups within Afghanistan, for example, the Taliban. These conflicts can be quagmires, rife with a lot of "the enemy of my enemy is my friend" thinking, which leads to confusing, twisted alliances and unclear political off-ramps. As a result, they tend to last longer and involve more civilian deaths, and are much harder to settle by brute force.

The good news is that you don't have to understand these underlying complexities to recognize what fragile and conflict-affected states are. The World Bank publishes an annual list of fragile situations, and these are the states I will use as my standard as I discuss the health effects of fragility and conflict. More than one billion people live in fragile states (2021). While action to reduce conflict is demanded—if only from a moral imperative to support vulnerable people—we must also be realistic in knowing that tragedy doesn't respect borders. If hundreds of millions of people who simply happened to be born in Venezuela or Afghanistan or

Somalia, rather than in Switzerland or New Zealand or Japan, are left living in absolute desperation, not only will these crises continue to dominate global humanitarian efforts and prevent aid from being allocated to other important issues like climate change, but we will also see an increase in overall global political fragility. We are already seeing hints of this, such as the nationalist backlashes directed at refugees flowing into Europe or asylum-seekers into the United States.

There has been much debate about what to do with the refugees, what forms they should be required to fill out, how they should dress, and what language they should speak. There is much less discussion about addressing the circumstances that led them to make the intensely personal and difficult choice to leave their homelands.

THE VIOLENCE OF WAR IS POLITICAL

Even a cursory understanding of war brings to mind some pretty obvious health consequences. Bombs, guns, land mines, and chemical weapons kill and disable civilian populations, and we do our best to count these deaths and to identify the perpetrators and their victims. But we know that's not all there is. Many fragile and conflict-affected states are classified as low-income countries, which means that their health systems, even prior to conflict, were likely already lacking the capacity to provide basic services. Civilians living in fragile and conflict-affected states report a life expectancy almost 10 years lower than the global average (62.2 years and 71.4 years, respectively). Immunization rates are lower, risk factors for noncommunicable diseases are more prevalent, and rates of mental health distress are significantly higher (WHO, 2017).

We will dig into the details of these and many other health indicators, but for now, consider an infant boy who is brought to a hospital by his grandmothers after both of his parents are injured in a bombing. The grandmothers learn that the unpaid medical staff of the hospital walked out in protest on the previous day, after a guard working for the private security firm tasked with protecting the facility from militants assaulted one of the physicians. The grandmothers attempt to place the baby in an incubator themselves, but two of the machines were damaged in a recent bombing and were never fixed, due to blockades of needed imports. By the time they get the infant into a functional machine, the boy, Kenan, is dead. This story was featured in the *Washington Post*, but many similar ones happen every day, with little or no fanfare, only to be carried forever as a private burden by whoever lives on. They are left to consider whether they are the lucky ones who survived—or the unlucky ones, burdened to remember.

This single child's experience includes elements of all the weaknesses of health care in fragile and conflict-affected states with both direct and structural violence. First, bombing has directly hurt the child's family, and damaged any infrastructure that might have been able to provide lifesaving care. The hospital staff was unpaid, as so many in these environments are, working around the clock and experiencing high trauma themselves in settings with little chance of providing good outcomes for their patients. Corruption and power imbalances have led to unregulated private security firms offering protection when the state cannot. A blockade of the civilian population has kept damaged health care resources from being repaired. In the end, a child has died from what may have been an entirely preventable or treatable health condition: due to the mere fluke of when and where the boy happened to be born, he never stood a chance.

THE HUMANITARIAN RESPONSE TO WAR IS POLITICAL

The presence of humanitarian aid in war is as ubiquitous as war itself. Global agencies like the International Committee of the Red Cross (ICRC) and the International Rescue Committee (IRC), along with thousands of grassroots organizations, spend billions of dollars in donor funds every year to maintain some semblance of access to basic social services, such as health care and education, and to reduce human suffering. Of these billions of dollars spent on overall humanitarian aid, conflict is the primary driver of global humanitarian need. The OECD estimates that in 2016, donors to fragile and conflict-affected states provided nearly $70 billion in aid; however, only 10% of that aid went to peacebuilding efforts, and only 2% went to conflict prevention (2018). This suggests that globally, while we are spending billions of dollars to ensure that people receive aid, we are doing much less to address the reasons for the conflict, or of state fragility, both root causes of people needing aid to begin with.

Additionally, donor behavior is swayed by domestic politics and other pressures, and may not be the most effective means of providing a path for long-term health system building. Donors active in the conflict phase, or immediately after the conflict ceases, may start to pull their aid a few years into the "post-conflict" period—right when fragile states need the most support to maintain stability. Generally, a few high-priority, or high-profile, crises tend to receive the greatest amount of aid, leaving other fragile and conflict-affected nations to work with much less.

Despite the billions of aid dollars spent, almost all fragile and conflict-affected states receive significantly less than what is needed to make significant impacts in long-term capacity. Most aid projects are piecemeal efforts, intended to deal with a specific need, leaving efforts uncoordinated and not as effective as when efforts are pooled where need is greatest. Lastly, often the government officials of fragile and conflict-affected states are not the best arbiters of what to do with large sums of largely unaccountable funds. They might not apply the aid to where it is needed most, do little to support civil society efforts, or waste the aid due to inefficient projects or corruption.

While it cannot be denied that, in areas experiencing extreme poverty, famine, and public health crises, humanitarian aid does alleviate the worst of outcomes, many scholars are critical of the current models of aid deployment. They cite depression of local economies, political (rather than humanitarian) motivations, and the tendency for aid to ease the pressure on warring parties to look for political settlements, by alleviating the worst of humanitarian outcomes. In allocating aid, donors tend to favor states that are small, close, and/or less politically divisive. Further, a "bandwagon" effect can occur, where donors are likely to donate only after other major donors have contributed (Fink & Redaelli, 2011).

What does this mean? While billions in aid dollars flow around the globe, donors don't necessarily consider who needs the aid most, or the best ways to spend it in the places that do need it. No one wants to turn down money to build a new clinic, or to say no to a vaccination effort, even if these aren't the local health priorities or sustainable in the long-term. It is hard to contend with humanitarian models of response that are inefficient and/or subject to political pressures, with stakeholders unable to respond directly with best practices to improve health outcomes on the ground.

Of course, the type of war and form of warfare employed also dictate the scope and type of humanitarian response. For instance, a drone attack on a single facility housing a terrorist cell in a desolate desert region would garner almost no humanitarian intervention, assuming no civilians were harmed in the attack. On the other end of the spectrum, the almost complete destruction of cities by bombs dropped by state militaries, the use of chemical weapons, and such secondary outcomes as starvation, would require a massive intervention; not just of humanitarian capacity but also all the logistical support needed to rebuild physical infrastructure.

The length of the conflict, the type of actors involved and their motivations, and the quality of social services that were in place before the conflict began are also important factors to weigh when deploying humanitarian resources in a fragile environment. Yemen, for example, was already one of the poorest and least-served countries on earth prior to the beginning of the current war in 2015, and Saudi Arabia's use of state-sponsored attacks has only increased the destruction on the ground. The role of Saudi Arabia, an economically important nation with generally good ties with the global community, as the primary antagonist has also complicated the cessation of the conflict and the need for humanitarian intervention. This is a prime, and quite recent, example of politics dictating not only the lethality of the conflict, but the world's humanitarian response—or lack thereof.

REFERENCES

Berchick, E., & Mykyta, L. (2019, September 10). *Children's public health insurance coverage lower than in 2017.* US Census Bureau. https://census.gov/library /stories/2019/09/uninsured-rate-for-children-in-2018.html.

Blanton, R., Mason, T., Athow, B. (2001). Colonial style and post-colonial ethnic conflict in Africa. *Journal of Peace Research, 38*(4), 473–491.

Brodie, B. (1973). *War and politics.* New York: Macmillan.

Bruhn, M., & Gallego, F. (2012). Good, bad, and ugly colonial activities: do they matter for economic development? *The Review of Economics and Statistics, 94*(2), 433–461.

Carville, O. (2018). The super rich of Silicon Valley have a doomsday escape plan. *Bloomberg.* https://www.bloomberg.com/features/2018-rich-new-zealand -doomsday-preppers/#xj4y7vzkg.

Cirillo, P., & Taleb, N. N. (2016). On the statistical properties and tail risk of violent conflicts. *Physica A: Statistical Mechanics and Its Applications, 452,* 29–45.

Crawford, N. (2019). *United States budgetary costs and obligations of post-9/11 wars through FY2020: $6.4 trillion.* Watson Institute. https://watson.brown.edu /costsofwar/files/cow/imce/papers/2019/US%20Budgetary%20Costs%20 of%20Wars%20November%202019.pdf.

Del Sarto, R. (2017). Contentious borders in the Middle East and North Africa. *International Affairs, 93*(4), 767–787.

Development Initiatives. (2019). *Global humanitarian assistance report 2019.* http://devinit.org/wp-content/uploads/2019/09/GHA-report-2019.pdf.

Engerman, S., & Sokoloff, K. (2005). Colonialism, inequality, and long-run paths of development. (NBER working paper no. 11057). National Bureau of Economic Research. https://www.nber.org/papers/w11057.pdf.

Falk, D., & Hildebolt, C. (2017). Annual war deaths in small-scale versus state societies scale with population size rather than violence. *Current Anthropology, 58*(6), 805–813.

Fanon, F. (1961). *The wretched of the earth.* New York: Grove Press.

Fink, G., & Redaelli, S. (2011). Determinants of international emergency aid— humanitarian need only? *World Development, 39*(5), 741–757.

Global Burden of Disease 2015 Maternal Mortality Collaborators. (2016). Global, regional, and national levels of maternal mortality, 1990–2015: a systematic analysis for the Global Burden of Disease Study 2015. *Lancet, 388,* 1775–1812.

International Physicians for the Prevention of Nuclear War (IPPNW). (n.d.). *IPPNW: a brief history.* Retrieved from https://www.ippnw.org/about/ippnw-a -brief-history.

Iqbal, M., Bardwell, H., & Hammond, D. (2019). Estimating the global economic cost of violence: methodology improvement and estimate updates. *Defence and Peace Economics.* https://doi.org/10.1080/10242694.2019.1689485.

Lasker, J. (1977). The role of health services in colonial rule: the case of the Ivory Coast. *Culture, Medicine and Psychiatry, 1,* 277–297.

Magone, C., Neuman, M., & Weissman, F. (2012). *Humanitarian negotiations revealed: the MSF experience.* Retrieved from https://www.msf-crash.org/en/publications/humanitarian-negotiations-revealed-msf-experience.

Manderson, L. (1987). Health services and legitimation of the colonial state: British Malaya 1786-1941. *International Journal of Health Services, 17*(1), 91-112.

Nathan, D., Geiger, H., Sidel, V., & Lown, B. (1962). The medical consequences of thermonuclear war. *The New England Journal of Medicine, 266*(22), 1126-1127.

Organisation for Economic Co-operation and Development (OECD). (2019). *Social spending (indicator).* https://doi.org/10.1787/7497563b-en.

Oka, R., Kissel, M., Golitko, M., Sheridan, S., Kim, N., & Fuentes, A. (2017). Population is the main driver of war group size and conflict casualties. *Proceedings of the National Academy of Sciences, 114*(52), E11101-E11110.

Orbinski, J. (1999). *The Nobel Peace Prize speech.* Médecins Sans Frontières. https://www.msf.org/ru/node/19856.

Sidel, V., Geiger, H., & Lown, B. (1962). The physician's role in the postattack period. *The New England Journal of Medicine, 266*(22), 1137-1145.

Strand, H., Rustad, S., Urdal, H., & Nygard, H. (2019). *Trends in armed conflict, 1946-2018.* Peace Research Institute Oslo. https://www.prio.org/utility/DownloadFile.ashx?id=1858&type=publicationfile.

Turshen, M. (1977). The impact of colonialism on health and health services in Tanzania. *International Journal of Health Services, 7*(1), 7-35.

Waitzkin, H. (2000). *The second sickness: contradictions of capitalist health care.* Lanham, MD: Rowman & Littlefield.

World Bank. (2021). *Population, total—fragile and conflict affected situations.* https://data.worldbank.org/indicator/SP.POP.TOTL?locations=F1.

CHAPTER 3

COLLECTIVE DIRECT VIOLENCE

As long as they killed people with conventional rather than nuclear weapons, they were praised as humanitarian statesmen. As long as they did not use nuclear weapons, it appeared, nobody was going to give the right name to all the killing that had been going on since the end of the Second World War, which was surely "World War Three."

—KURT VONNEGUT, *Galápagos* (1985)

Hand guns are made for killin'
They ain't no good for nothin' else.

—LYNYRD SKYNYRD, "Saturday Night Special" (1975)

THE SCHÖNINGEN SPEARS ARE THE OLDEST preserved weapons in the archeological record, thought to have been crafted in the Paleolithic Age at least 300,000 years ago. Several of the spears—sleek and aerodynamic, with a pointed tip—show signs of being projectile weapons, while the other, stouter ones were likely designed for thrusting at shorter distances. Traces of smoothing and sharpening can be seen, indicating they were used multiple times. Some were found among the remains of butchered horses, including one still sticking out of a horse's pelvis. These rudimentary weapons, just thin tree trunks that were stripped and shaped, were used by humans' predecessors, potentially *Homo heidelbergensis* or even early Neanderthals, to hunt (Schoch, Bigga, Böhner, Richter, & Terberger, 2015). They were developed to provide food and defend against attacks from large animals. They were used, ultimately, to sustain and protect life.

Hundreds of thousands of years later, evidence of a wholly different use for weaponry has been unearthed at many ancient sites. For millions of years, our ancestors were hunter-gatherers, dependent on foraging for wild plants and killing prey without getting killed. Evidence suggests that these populations were nomadic and lived in small groups, which makes sense: you need to be able to easily pick up and leave when local food sources dwindle, if you don't know how to produce your own; and a large and unruly group would make that difficult.

There is some lively debate about what life was like during these long periods, from which precious little evidence remains. However, what we do understand is that, as hunter-gatherer societies learned how to cultivate and store crops and to tend to animals, they shifted from small, nomadic groups to settled agrarian societies. Looking at where they started and where we are today, it is almost impossible to comprehend just how many tiny individual decisions and random accidents had to accrue, over countless years, for us to end up in a world with New York City and global supply chains and satellites.

These early peoples developed small settlements with farms. Different roles had to be assigned to different residents to keep things running. Eventually, they built canals and dams to divert water, figured out what to do with waste, and developed methods for storing food to keep it from spoiling or being eaten by animals. Eventually, a system is created, and value is aggregated. With it comes power and a sense of ownership: *This is the land and these are the resources that belong to our group.* No longer struggling just to survive, they find that competition, domination, and exploitation are possible. Protecting people and resources becomes a priority; we start to see settlements with walls and other physical barriers. And of course, the development of weapons far beyond sharpened sticks.

The first firearm is thought to have emerged from the Song Dynasty in China almost 1,200 years ago. Gunpowder was attached to the shafts of arrows and ignited, shooting the arrows long distances. Eventually, gunpowder traveled to Europe, probably through trade routes. Cannons were developed, then hand cannons. As Europeans crossed the Atlantic to settle in the New World, they brought their shotguns and muskets with them. In the eighteenth and nineteenth centuries, the development of revolvers and machine guns evolved quickly. Through needs spurred by multiple wars and aggressive territorial expansion, weapons were crafted to suit the moment with the latest available technology. In this way, the trajectory of weapons follows a course not unrelated to our development as societies, complete with organizing principles and hierarchies that we would recognize today.

That is not to say there was no inter-group violence prior to settlement. At Jebel Sahaba in the Nile River Valley, a cemetery was discovered in the 1960s that has been dated to be 13,400 to 18,600 years old; it contains what has widely been cited as the earliest evidence of organized warfare. Dozens of bodies with various injuries—from blunt-force trauma to penetrative wounds from projectiles like light or heavy arrows and spears—were found, many with signs of healed injuries that indicate previous violence. The use of projectile weapons suggests that these were inter-group conflicts, not conflicts within the group. Yet, scientists are undecided whether this signifies a single conflict or if the burial site was designated for those injured over a longer period of time (Crevecoeur et al., 2021).

Another site that appears to offer evidence of inter-group violence between hunter-gatherers was found in Nataruk, Kenya, and is about 10,000 years old. More than two dozen bodies, including those of children and a pregnant woman, were discovered in what amounted to a mass grave. The bodies showed significant and deliberate damage from what appear to be arrow wounds and blunt force trauma, and evidence suggests that some of the victims were bound when killed (Lahr et al., 2016). As with Jebel Sahaba, some scholars dispute that there exists enough evidence to consider these bodies victims of inter-group violence at all, although there is broad agreement that violence was present among hunter-gatherer populations (Stojanowski, Seidel, Fulginiti, Johnson, & Buikstra, 2016).

What happened at Jebel Sahaba or Nataruk? We don't know, and probably never will. It is often said that violence and warfare are inherent aspects of human nature, and these early violent events seem to bear that out. But even though we can't know for sure what happened, most historians and anthropologists maintain that these early instances of violence most likely resulted from conflict over land and resources. The use of direct collective violence to achieve a political or economic end has remained consistent for many thousands of years, ever since our far-distant ancestors first realized that violence was a potent tool to get what they wanted. You could threaten harm; you could harm; if necessary, you could kill. These principles haven't changed. The instruments we use to wage this violence, especially on a large scale, have changed significantly. But the purpose hasn't.

Collective violence is the term for violence between groups to achieve political, social, or economic goals (WHO, 2002). As with any threat to health, it is vital to understand the mechanisms of potential harm and how they work; think of a cigarette, an infectious pathogen, or contaminated water pipes. In science, we rely on evidence: in the case of war, this includes the weapons and the ways those weapons are used on the population level. Collective direct violence is not possible without weaponry. Physical trauma is a fundamental public health threat during war, one that affects civilians and combatants alike; but we can't fully understand it until we understand the weapons that make it possible.

While modern weapons make the task simple, the purpose of the harm caused by these weapons is complex. The goal of the belligerent actor may be any number of things: to terrorize populations and induce compliance; to induce fear in local populations and those who hear of the violence; to push leaders to acquiesce to settlement; to motivate migration from desired areas; or simply to reduce the number of people on the opposing side who are left alive and fighting. Of course, the belligerent actor's motivations may also be rooted in a psychological need, including vengeance and dehumanization.

Physical attacks also serve as a show of power, mimicking the tactics of a typical abuser: *Look what I can do, and look at how powerless you are. Look what I can do—don't make me do it again.* Although based on the ways we've been hurting and killing each other for millennia, today's weapons are far more efficient than weapons from even a century ago. If science fiction has taught us anything, it's that this is not a promising development. That said, it's important to consider the lethal tools of today, and their effects on the body.

CONVENTIONAL WEAPONS

Perhaps no weapon is more associated with war than the tank. Unlike guns, planes, or drones, there is no civilian use for a tank—a tank is a heavily armored machine, designed only for war. A tank is visceral—loud, destructive, literally shaking the ground, while emitting the obtrusive smell of diesel smoke. Its tracks allow it to maneuver in areas that might otherwise be untraversable. Most have a turret equipped with prominent, protruding cannons or guns that leave no question of its power or intention. What is this weapon, or any modern weapon, really, but technology crafted specifically to kill others?

The power differential couldn't be starker between the individuals in a tank—who are not visible, rendering the tank seemingly devoid of humanity—and those outside. One of the most famous images in recent history remains that of "Tank Man," the unknown Chinese man who stood before a line of approaching tanks in Tiananmen Square in Beijing, China, in 1989. This solitary man, holding mere shopping bags, used his own body to temporarily block the movement of these 30-ton behemoths, at one point even climbing onto the front tank and attempting to communicate with the crew through the hatch, perhaps even making contact (although no audio is available). What he may have said or didn't say, however, didn't matter. The act of facing near-certain death in such a standoff was a powerful show of bravery and defiance that worries an authoritarian regime dependent on submission. To face down a tank operated by an adversarial force is to openly face one's own mortality.

The United Nations (UN) designates "conventional weapons" to be all those that are not weapons of mass destruction. This includes tanks and other armored vehicles, artillery systems, combat aircraft, uncrewed combat aerial vehicles (better known as drones), warships, missiles, land mines, and small arms. These weapons, and their use, are legal when operated under the auspices of international law; but some conventional weapons, because of their indiscriminate nature (in other words, their ability to kill civilians just as easily as targeted combatants), are banned. These include anti-personnel land mines and cluster munitions, which randomly scatter munitions over a wide area.

From just the 25 largest corporations in the sector, conventional weapons make up a significant part of the $361 billion in arms sales and military services from 2019 alone. The top five companies are based in the United States, with almost half of the total in sales: Lockheed Martin, Boeing, Northrop Grumman, Raytheon, and General Dynamics. China took the second-largest share of arms sales, at 16%, Western European countries together accounted for 18%, and Russia comes in at about 4%. This represented an 8.5% increase from 2018 (SIPRI, 2020).

There are many global frameworks meant to regulate these weapons. The Programme of Action to Prevent, Combat and Eradicate the Illicit Trade in Small Arms and Light Weapons in All Its Aspects (PoA) was adopted in 2001, ensuring that small arms are properly marked, traced, and regulated. That same year, The Protocol against the Illicit Manufacturing of and Trafficking in Firearms, their Parts and Components and Ammunition was adopted to control the illicit manufacturing and trafficking of firearms. The Arms Trade Treaty was adopted by the UN General Assembly in 2013 to prevent illicit trade and diversion of these weapons, and there have been many more attempts to regulate or prohibit these weapons globally, as discussed in this chapter. So, we can and do learn to set boundaries for weapons use, as demonstrated by these and many other global regulatory frameworks for arms. But are they enough?

You may notice a few things about these frameworks. One, they are mostly quite recent. Two, most don't really do anything about the existence of these weapons in general, with the exception of weapons of mass destruction; they just aim to ensure they aren't manufactured or distributed illegally. And, less noticeably, not all countries have signed onto them. For example, only 100 countries have ratified or approved the Arms Trade Treaty; worse, many countries, including some of the world's most authoritarian or brutal regimes, have refused to ratify or sign onto any of these frameworks. Many claim they do not want to limit their country's ability to defend itself. Herein lies a core dilemma about weapons: everyone thinks their uses are justified. They're especially justified if wielded by someone in a uniform. Thus, one country's airstrikes are lauded, while another's may be condemned. Individuals who have the power to engage in conflict, whether non-state militia leaders or heads of state, are entirely convinced of their own justifications for their indiscriminate harming of civilians. Even today, countries that posture themselves as just and democratic may easily justify civilian deaths in other countries as "collateral damage." This phrasing diverts attention away from questions about the weapons used, the reasons for using them, and the trauma and destruction they caused.

Conventional weapons, and the damage they cause, are those most associated with modern warfare. Their task is simple: render traumatic injury or death to victims, and damage or destroy infrastructure. In that sense, they are highly successful, in that they are responsible for most battle-related death and trauma. Yet generally, their use is rationalized with far more grandiose rhetoric; for example, the claim that attacking or killing large swaths of people, combatants or not, is necessary in service of a just political goal. Many political leaders even publicly bemoan the need to engage in such brutal actions—if only their antagonist were not quite so uncivilized or impossible to reason with. Indeed, with the current rules of war as we accept them, these sentiments are the only way to justify what are, all too often, acts of collective punishment, resulting in massive trauma, death, and destruction.

Standard operating procedure dictates that violence must be met with violence, that military budgets must constantly be inflated, and that the most important form of security is that which can be promised by a new weapons system. In this way, possession, production, and use of conventional weapons can be construed as a symptom of the epidemic of war that spreads and infects countries and non-state actors at an exponential rate.

Below is a brief description of the conventional weapons that are most often associated with battle-related death and trauma.

BOMBS

"The bomb is the chief weapon of an air force and the principal means by which it may attain its aim in war," according to the 1936 Royal Air Force War Manual (Hall, 1998). Bombs, like tanks, are almost wholly associated with warfare or terrorism. Consumers of news articles and broadcasts about war are all too familiar with the images associated with these weapons in the public consciousness: decimated buildings and city blocks, children learning in destroyed classrooms with exposed rebar and crumbling cinder blocks, or the bloody aftermath of a crowded market that was attacked by a suicide bomber. They can range from homemade efforts (or improvised explosive devices, IEDs), such as the pressure cookers used by the Boston Marathon bombers, to, more commonly, ordnance produced and deployed by state militaries, like those used so widely by Bashar al-Assad in Syria. It's estimated that, between 2012 and 2021, the Syrian regime dropped 82,000 barrel bombs—containers filled with explosive material—that killed tens of thousands of Syrians. More than 60,000 of these bombs were dropped after the United Nations Security Council passed Resolution No. 2139, banning their use (Syrian Network for Human Rights, 2021).

Airstrikes—bombs dropped from the air—have existed for almost as long as planes, or even longer: there is evidence that in the mid-1800s, Austrians attempted to drop bombs on Venice from hot air balloons. Initially, bombs were dropped from planes freely, with the mere hope, often failed, of hitting their targets. Today, "smart" precision-guided bombs are supposed to minimize accidents and increase successful strikes. Bombs can also be specially designed for different actions for certain targets, like releasing a pressure wave upon impact to collapse a building.

Most military bombs are large metal casings with an explosive inside, designated by weight (commonly up to about 2,000 lbs.). IEDs are most often used by non-state actors because they don't have access to an air force or the necessary technology for general-purpose bombs. These improvised devices include pipe bombs, fertilizer truck bombs, and Molotov cocktails.

A Molotov cocktail is a homemade example of an incendiary weapon, which is meant to ignite upon impact, rather than detonate. These types of bombs, which for military purposes are filled with combustible chemicals like napalm, were banned in the 1980 Convention on Conventional Weapons (CCW) Protocol III on Incendiary Weapons, largely because of their widespread use by the American military during the Vietnam War. Because Vietnam was the first televised war, Americans saw the effects of these horrific bombings firsthand; and the effects of this "liquid fire" on the Vietnamese, including children, moved many Americans to protest. Martin Luther King Jr. declared, "When I see our country today intervening in what is basically a civil war, destroying hundreds of thousands of Vietnamese children with napalm, leaving broken bodies in countless fields . . . and all this in the name of pursuing the goal of peace—I tremble for our world" (1967).

There is also the reality that bombs often kill other people than their intended targets, sometimes as part of "collateral damage," but also due to outright mistakes or (less charitably) malice. In 2016, Saudi Arabia bombed a funeral in Yemen, killing 140 people and wounding 600, later blaming "wrong information" (*The Guardian*, 2016). In 2014, Israel dropped two bombs on four boys, aged 9-11, who were playing on the beach in the Gaza Strip, killing them all. They deemed the incident a "tragic accident" (Beaumont, 2015). The Nigerian Air Force killed at least 100 civilians, including 20 Red Cross workers, when it bombed a refugee camp in 2017. Their military commander claimed it was "too early to say if a tactical error was made" (AP, 2017). These are just a few of the unfortunately countless examples.

In Afghanistan between 2017 and 2020, the number of civilians killed in air strikes by the United States and allies increased by 330%; this followed a policy in which airstrikes were increased, made possible by the limited number of US troops on the ground. The Brown University Costs of War project (2020) notes that this epitomized the US premise that "air power works to coerce its enemies and bring them to the negotiating table," quoting a US general who claimed, "The entire purpose behind our air campaign is to pressure the Taliban into reconciliation and help them realize that peace talks are their best option." In retrospect, bombing a country to incentivize peace talks did not appear to be a successful strategy.

LAND MINES AND CLUSTER MUNITIONS

The cause of clearing land mines has led many anti-war efforts in recent decades. Land mines are explosive devices that are shallowly buried in the ground; this makes them especially problematic, since they are often planted haphazardly and without records, and so can linger long after a conflict has ended, causing sudden and indiscriminate death or injury years later. Although 164 countries adhere to the Mine Ban Treaty that was adopted in 1997, many of the largest military states, like China, India, Israel, Pakistan, Russia, and the United States, are not party to the treaty. From 2019 to 2020, Myanmar was the only government still known to use land mines. However, non-state actors in several other countries (Afghanistan, Colombia, India, Myanmar, and Pakistan) used anti-personnel mines during these years, and there were many unconfirmed uses elsewhere, including in Syria, Yemen, and Somalia.

In 2019, just over 2,000 people were killed and 3,000 injured by land mines and explosive remnants, 80% of whom were civilians (43% of them children). It's estimated that 55 million stockpiled anti-personnel mines have been destroyed by adherents to the Mine Ban Treaty, but 64 of these countries retain mines (for training and research), with Ukraine still possessing more than three million. Twelve states, including Russia, China, and the United States, have not guaranteed that they will not produce further land mines. At the same time, donors contributed $561.3 million to land mine actions in 2019, which includes clearance and victim assistance (International Campaign to Ban Landmines, 2020).

Although the method of deployment differs between land mines and cluster munitions, both are significant causes of indiscriminate harm to civilians. The latter, also called cluster bombs, are essentially large containers with smaller "bomblets" inside. As they are deployed, they open in midair to release up to 600 smaller submunitions. These are not individually guided, and so fall where they fall. Aside from being indiscriminate, they do not explode on impact 10–40% of the time, which means they stay on the ground, sometimes hidden, posing a long-term threat to civilians or humanitarian workers moving through affected areas.

During the Vietnam War, more than 270 million cluster bombs were dropped on Laos by the United States, making it the most heavily bombed country per capita; up to 80 million of these did not detonate. More than 20,000 Laotians have been killed by this unexploded ordnance since the end of the war, and 40% of these victims were children (Legacies of War, 2021). These weapons were prohibited in the 2008 Convention on Cluster Munitions, but dozens of countries still hold on to their stockpiles (ICRC, 2010).

FIREARMS, SMALL ARMS, GUNS

Firearms differ from land mines and bombs in that they must be deployed by one individual against another at relatively close quarters, with the rare exception of top sniper shooters, who can hit their targets from up to two miles away. That makes these weapons more personal and direct than bombs of any kind: someone must pull the trigger, with the full intention of inflicting, at the very least, severe pain and debilitation. Guns are also widely available in many countries, with an estimated one billion in circulation worldwide; they are easily available to many civilian populations, although not in the same caliber available to militaries. They can be easily transported, both legally and illicitly.

Most of the world's guns (85%) are thought to be in civilian hands, but since many countries don't release details of their stockpiles, it's impossible to be completely sure about the numbers. Though they predict a much higher number, the Small Arms Survey (2018), based on currently available information, estimates that the armed forces of 177 countries possess at least 133 million firearms combined. Firearm stockpiles are highly concentrated in just a few countries, and over 43% of these firearms belong to just two (Russia and China), while the top 10 countries together hold about 70%.

Almost three-quarters of these weapons are modern self-loading service rifles, or what are often referred to as assault rifles, like the AK-47. The M16A2/A4 assault rifle is the top weapon of the world's most powerful military—the United States Armed Forces—and more than eight million have been sold in more than 80 countries. But many similar guns are being produced for militaries around the world, like the K2 from South Korea and the AK-74 from Russia. These fully automatic, magazine-fed weapons are designed to keep shooting rounds as long as the trigger is held, and are not intended for civilian use, due to their potential for mass violence. Yet even in the intended hands, these weapons are incredibly dangerous, with a disturbing potential for so-called collateral damage. The 2016 US Army's Rifle and Carbine Training Circular warns that "Automatic and burst fires drastically decrease the probability of hit due to the rapid succession of recoil impulses and the inability of the Soldier to maintain proper sight alignment and sight picture on the target."

UNCREWED AERIAL VEHICLES, A.K.A. DRONES

Drones are among the newest entrants to the battlefield, and their selling points are simple. They are operated remotely, so no personnel need be put in direct danger through their operation. The drone strike operator does not even have to be in the field—they can wake up at home, go to work and manage their drone, and then return to the safety of their home. Drones can more easily reach difficult-to-access areas than can crewed weaponry, and most drones held by militaries are not armed and are used only for surveillance. When armed, they are marketed as a more precise, even humane, way to kill targets while minimizing civilian casualties. Many early drone strikes were conducted in remote areas, however, where there was little chance of anyone investigating whether all of the victims were truly terrorists, as was always claimed.

Drones raise many legal and ethical questions, most of which have not been properly adjudicated since their relatively recent inception. In 2013, US President Barack Obama was criticized for targeting a US citizen, Anwar al-Awlaki, in a drone strike in Yemen. The same strike also killed three other US citizens; and a month later, al-Awlaki's 16-year-old son, also a US citizen, was killed by yet another drone strike (Taylor, 2015).

The United States was among the first to acquire armed drones, in the early 2000s, conducting the first drone strikes in Afghanistan during the post-9/11 invasion. It is estimated that today, about 39 countries have armed drones—with the United States, Israel, and China among the top producers—but less than a third have actually carried out strikes (Bergen, Salyk-Virk, & Sterman, 2020). Drones are becoming increasingly popular in military budgets due to their purported strengths, but the reality seems murkier. As one special operations source told *The Intercept* (Scahill, 2015) about the plight of potential drone targets: "They have no rights. They have no dignity. They have no humanity to themselves. . . . Anyone caught in the vicinity is guilty by association."

During the withdrawal from Afghanistan in 2021, a US drone, in what was initially alleged to be a "righteous strike," targeted an Iraqi worker for a US aid organization who was bringing home canisters of water for his family. The strike killed 10 people in all, including seven children (Aikins, Koettl, Hill, & Schmitt, 2021). "It was a tragic mistake," the Pentagon stated in a press conference, once the *New York Times* had reported that their initial recounting was false.

One analysis claims that tens of thousands of civilians have been killed by US drone strikes alone. However, it is impossible to know for sure, since this data is extremely difficult to collect and verify; and most state actors won't willingly admit failures without supporting evidence, especially videos. The first drone strike carried out by the United States, way back in 2001, was meant to kill Mullah Mohammad Omar, the supreme leader of the Taliban. It missed. In fact, drone strikes targeting Omar missed their target for many more years, killing many others in the process. Eventually, Omar died of natural causes (Feroz, 2021).

Aside from their potential to cause deadly harm with little accountability, drones may change the cost-benefit calculation of those who possess them, especially as they become cheaper and more effective. When you don't have to invest in the logistics of traveling to and safely infiltrating a location to capture or assassinate a target, with the assumption that several of your own personnel may die, you can afford to take risks with others' lives that you might not otherwise take. And when you don't have people on the ground doing background work on potential targets, there is a greater likelihood of a mistaken identity. Lastly, emerging research suggests that because drones are so much cheaper than many other weapons, both financially and in terms of potential friendly lives lost, adversaries can afford to keep wars going longer (Zegart, 2020).

LESS-LETHAL WEAPONS

Although most often produced for domestic police and security forces, the use of what are colloquially called "non-lethal" weapons, long used by oppressive regimes against civilian protests and other gatherings, has increasingly been the target of scrutiny by the public health community. These weapons—e.g., rubber bullets, bean bag rounds, pepper spray, tasers, tear gas and skunk gas; and devices that use light, sound, or heat to incapacitate victims—are supposed to be used for crowd control, offering protection for security details, convoys, and other sensitive transport (Pan, 2005). They're often called non-lethal, but they can, and do, injure and kill. A 2017 study of available information about incidents since 1990 found that of 1,984 affected people, 53 died and 300 suffered permanent disability, primarily from rubber and plastic bullets (Haar, Iacopino, Ranadive, Dandu, & Weiser, 2017).

Companies produce these types of weapons both for domestic law enforcement and for security forces in countries with histories of human rights violations, like Egypt, Colombia, Israel, and Bahrain. Demand is increasing throughout the world, including from the US Department of Defense. The global market for these weapons was $7.4 billion in 2020, and is estimated to reach more than $12 billion by 2028. Most are produced in the United States, with other major producers in Brazil, Germany, and Israel (Joshi & Mutreja, 2021). In the US, these companies are often situated in towns facing economic downturns, with lax regulations and workers in need of jobs. One company built their headquarters in rural Jamestown, Pennsylvania, in 1995; they replaced ponds and fields with firing ranges and manufacturing plants. Soon, families in nearby houses complained about the constant explosions, waves of tear gas wafting over toward their homes, and multiple fires, not to mention hundreds of munitions, many live, strewn throughout the woods. One homeowner who sued the company claimed it amounted to psychological torture, saying, "Living next door, you have a very real experience of what other people go through. And it just shouldn't be used. Period. On any-body, for any reason" (Sands, 2021).

WEAPONS OF MASS DESTRUCTION

"Simply stated, there is no doubt that Saddam Hussein now has weap-ons of mass destruction," Vice President Dick Cheney told the world in 2002 (*The Guardian*, 2002). We know now, and Cheney and many others likely knew at the time, that this was not true. Yet he and the other mem-bers of the Bush administration ushered the phrase "Weapons of Mass Destruction" into our everyday lexicon. Weapons of Mass Destruction (WMD) are those that can lead to mass and indiscriminate casualties and/ or destruction of infrastructure: typically nuclear, chemical, and biologi-cal weapons. They are the weapons most feared and most restricted, because of the potential for significant harm, especially (potentially) in the hands of terrorist groups, who typically show little hesitation in inflict-ing significant civilian casualties.

CHEMICAL AND BIOLOGICAL WEAPONS

Syria's government had already shocked the world in many ways by 2012, just a year after protests against the repressive regime had broken out on the heels of the Arab Spring and the Syrian government responded with massive violent force. Yet, four months after President Obama issued his infamous "red-line" speech prohibiting the use of chemical weapons in Syria, reports came out of Homs, Syria, that a poisonous gas, later iden-tified as Agent 15, was used to kill at least seven people on December 23. On March 19, 2013, another incident was reported, this time killing at least 25 and injuring many more. The Syrian government did not deny that chemical weapons were used but blamed the Syrian opposition for the attack. Over the coming years, many more allegations of the use of chemical weapons in Syria came to light, including sarin gas, chlorine gas, and VX gas, with international bodies prompting multiple investigations and, ultimately, finding sufficient evidence that chemical weapons were used, and that the Assad regime was responsible. These attacks continued even after Syria agreed to dispose of, destroy, or transfer all its chemical weapon stores by January 31, 2014 (Arms Control Association, 2021b).

Chemical weapons are poisonous substances, typically in gas form, that injure or kill their victims through toxic effects on the skin, lungs, nerves, or other parts of the body. Many of the substances used to produce these weapons have traditional uses, including crop fertilization or the production of plastics. Although banned for military purposes, confirmed use of these substances has recurred throughout the twentieth century, perhaps most famously by the United States in the Vietnam War, where the herbicide Agent Orange was sprayed by US Air Force jets over wide swaths of Vietnam. While the stated purpose was just to kill the vegetation used for cover by the Vietcong, millions of Vietnamese people were exposed and continue to suffer long-term health effects (von Meding, 2017).

Biological weapons, on the other hand, use microorganisms—viruses, bacteria, and fungi—to deliberately cause harm to living beings. The most infamous example is probably anthrax, which is a spore-forming bacterium that can cause serious injury or death. There has not been a confirmed use of biological weapons by state actors since World War I, despite various antagonists accusing each other in wartime, and the (false) belief of some that viruses like HIV and even COVID-19 were deployed as biological weapons. That said, many countries maintain biological weapons programs, purportedly for research and testing purposes.

Chemical and biological weapons were banned after World War I. Further bans in 1972 and 1993 prohibited their development, stockpiling, and transfer (ICRC, 2013). While the existence of chemical weapons stores have been confirmed in the United States, Russia, and Iraq, no countries have admitted to maintaining offensive biological weapons programs. According to US intelligence, however, some countries, including South Africa, Israel, and Iraq, may have just such programs (Frischknecht, 2003). While rarely deployed, these weapons, considered the "poor man's nuclear bomb," are thought by analysts to pose the greatest potential threat to human life, due to their relatively cheap and easy production process, not to mention the entirely indiscriminate dissemination of its lethal agents.

NUCLEAR WEAPONS

What is any discussion of the weapons of war without Hiroshima and Nagasaki? They were the only two sites of the offensive use of nuclear weapons after the technology was developed in 1942 by the Manhattan Project team. Once the possibility of splitting the atom—whereby huge amounts of energy are released in a chain reaction—became a reality, the scientist who first conceived of it, Leo Szilard, reportedly said, "This will go down as a black day in the history of mankind" (*New Scientist*, n.d.). In fact, many of the scientists who worked on the project are thought to have been morally opposed to it, but nevertheless continued their work, out of fear that the Nazis would develop the technology first—a fear ultimately discovered to be unfounded.

The scientists' fears of the technology's use, however, were well founded. The Japanese attacked Pearl Harbor in December 1941, and the US decision to react came quickly. Less quickly came the decision on how. Although then-President Franklin Roosevelt immediately called for retaliatory conventional bombing campaigns in Japan, the distance of the island nation from the nearest land base available to American planes meant that a full-scale invasion of Japan would be expensive and likely cost many American lives. In July 1945, upon receiving word that the first nuclear bomb test in New Mexico had been successful, Roosevelt's successor Harry Truman reportedly wrestled with the decision of whether to deploy the weapon in Japan. We all know what he decided. On August 6, 1945, the first uranium bomb detonated over Hiroshima, damaging or destroying 70% of the city and causing more than 100,000 deaths. Three days later, an even larger plutonium bomb was dropped on Nagasaki, killing approximately 70,000. While many who were at ground zero died immediately, many others succumbed in the coming days and years, mostly from radiation sickness and lack of care, as most medical personnel were killed and facilities destroyed by the blast (ICAN, 2021). Mere days after the bombing of Nagasaki, the emperor of Japan forced the military leaders to surrender.

The atomic bombs are thought to mark the official end of World War II, which was an undeniably brutal war for so many. Yet they also opened a Pandora's Box we have yet to close. A global arms race ensued, and the nature and expectation of military use evolved. The Cold War with the Soviet Union propelled development of weapons even more powerful than the atomic bombs used in Japan. A series of proxy wars between the United States and the Soviet Union accelerated conflicts and destabilized countries around the world, from Vietnam to Afghanistan to Cuba. Billions of dollars were squandered on building up military prowess, ostensibly to prevent another world war. It inspired President Dwight Eisenhower, a retired five-star Army general, to give his famous "military-industrial complex" farewell address in 1961, warning of America's increasing dependence on a standing military around the world and its addiction to ever-more sophisticated weaponry. "We must learn how to compose differences not with arms, but with intellect and decent purpose," he implored. Alas, we did not.

Although the United States was the first to develop the technology for nuclear weapons, conducted the first tests, and was the first and only power to use nuclear weapons in warfare, it did not long remain the only state to possess these highly destructive weapons. The Treaty on the Non-Proliferation of Nuclear Weapons was signed in 1968 and made permanent in 1995, and 191 states have joined the treaty, more than for any other arms agreement. At the same time, according to the Arms Control Association (2021a), there are still, as of October 2021, more than 13,000 nuclear warheads in the world, including about 3,500 that are "retired." More than 90% are held by the United States (5,550) and Russia (6,255), followed by China (350), France (290), the UK (225), Pakistan (165), India (156), Israel (90), and North Korea (estimated to have enough material for about 40–50).

CRIMES AGAINST HUMANITY AND GENOCIDE

Crimes against humanity—you don't have to be a legal or political expert to understand the meaning of such a phrase. These crimes are the worst of the worst, entailing the most egregious, senseless, and brutal violence.

They are not specific to any particular weapon or form of violence, or even any particular type of actor; they can be committed by a government, a non-state group, or an individual. The United States Institute of Peace defines them as "acts such as murder, extermination, enslavement, deportation, torture, rape, and disappearance, when committed as part of a widespread or systematic attack directed against any civilian population" (2008).

Because of the nature of these crimes and of the actors most likely to perpetrate them, it's difficult to get accurate data about the incidence of any of them, even when there is evidence that they occurred. While these crimes are not unique to any country, their perpetuation on a massive scale is typically limited to the war environment, where they are overtly used as tools of war and involve direct violence.

Torture is defined in the 1984 Convention against Torture and Other Cruel, Inhuman or Degrading Treatment or Punishment as "any act by which severe pain or suffering, whether physical or mental, is intentionally inflicted on a person for such purposes as obtaining from him or a third person information or a confession, punishing him for an act he or a third person has committed or is suspected of having committed, or intimidating or coercing him or a third person, or for any reason based on discrimination of any kind, when such pain or suffering is inflicted by or at the instigation of or with the consent or acquiescence of a public official or other person acting in an official capacity." Torture methods are diverse and often specific to certain groups or states. They can include waterboarding, overloading victims with light or sound, tying up detainees in uncomfortable and unnatural positions, neglecting medical needs of detainees, beatings, and application of electric shocks.

Significant evidence of torture has emerged from around the world, including China, Egypt, Indonesia, Iran, Iraq, Israel, Morocco, Nigeria, Pakistan, and Russia (Amnesty International, 2005). In the aftermath of 9/11, the United States lifted many prohibitions against torture and also implemented systematic and well-documented policies of torture, often euphemistically called "enhanced interrogation" programs and techniques (PHR, 2021). The country with the most reports of torture—as well as many of the other worst crimes against humanity that occur today—is Syria, where it is estimated that 13,197 people died due to torture between March 2011 and June 2018, including 167 children and 59 women, most at the hands of the Syrian regime (SNHR, 2018).

Unjust incarceration is certainly not limited to the war environment, but there is no doubt that imprisonment is a preferred tool for oppressive and belligerent regimes. An estimated 11 million people languish in prisons worldwide, with the United States holding nearly 20%, followed by China, Brazil, India, and Russia (World Prison Brief, 2021). About three million of them have not been convicted of any crime, or even had a trial. Amnesty International (2021) has outlined several issues with global detention and incarceration systems, many of which are highly relevant to the conflict-affected environment, including the detainment of prisoners of conscience, arbitrary detention, being detained without access to communication, secret detention, unfair trials, poor prison conditions, and poor treatment, including torture.

GENOCIDE AND ETHNIC CLEANSING

Over a period of four months in 1994, an estimated 400,000–800,000 people were murdered in Rwanda. On April 6, 1994, decades into an ethnic conflict, a plane carrying the president of Rwanda, a member of the Hutu ethnic majority, was shot down. Hutu actors blamed Tutsi political groups for the incident and used it to justify a campaign of mass murder against the Tutsi, calling for the Hutus to "weed out the cockroaches." Those identified as Tutsi were subject to summary execution, usually along with their families, by Hutu militias, who also kidnapped Tutsi women and subjected them to sexual abuse and violence. This violence from soldiers is, unfortunately, not historically unprecedented. But what seemed different about Rwanda was the murders of many Tutsis by ordinary people: their Hutu spouses, neighbors, teachers, vendors, even priests. The aim was clear: exterminate the Tutsi. Not for any purported individual crime, but merely due to their personal identity. This is genocide.

Genocide (*genos-* from the Latin for race or tribe, and *-cide* for killing) was not defined as a term until the 1948 Convention on the Prevention and Punishment of the Crime of Genocide, in light of the Nazi regime's explicit goals of extermination in the Holocaust. As such, genocide is defined as "acts committed with intent to destroy, in whole or in part, a national, ethnical, racial or religious group," and is only possible, by definition, as an act of collective violence.

Despite genocide being universally understood as among the worst possible acts, the international community has not meaningfully responded in any way to most instances of systematic mass murder in the past century. Even during the Holocaust, concentration camps existed for years prior to the US entrance into the war in 1941 upon the bombing of Pearl Harbor. Despite a long-standing belief that the extent of the Nazis' aims to exterminate Jews was unknown at the time, American newspapers had actually reported on Hitler and Nazi Germany's treatment of Jews and other groups throughout the 1930s; it just didn't register as a national priority worthy of military intervention (Bernstein, 1988). This belies the narrative that countries must maintain significant weapons stockpiles and hawkish postures to save the lives of innocents; when given the opportunity, most states with the military and political might to intervene choose not to.

In recent years, the codification of genocide as a crime has actually limited our ability to label violent acts as genocide and prosecute them as such, since they must fit a narrow legal definition that includes evidence of the full intent of the perpetrator, which is very difficult to prove (UN, 2021b). Accordingly, the term has only been applied to a few events outside of the Holocaust; examples include the Armenian genocide, in which the Ottoman Empire killed nearly 1.5 million people from 1915 to 1922 (at least three-quarters of the Armenian population), and the killing of nearly 500,000 ethnic Darfuris in Western Sudan by the Sudanese government in concert with paramilitary groups, which began in 2003. In all these instances, countless more victims were injured, abused, or displaced.

While genocide is a legal term that is meant to make a legal and political statement, many political stakeholders have been loath to use it against state actors, because it triggers accountability mechanisms that may strain political alliances; and it is always difficult to prove the intent to destroy a particular group, even if all actions point in that direction.

This means that actual convictions of states or non-state groups for genocide are incredibly rare; the prosecution of individuals affiliated with such groups is much more feasible. In 2021, for example, a German court found a former member of ISIS guilty of genocide and crimes against humanity for the murder of a five-year-old Yazidi girl in 2014. ISIS had made their genocidal claims against the Yazidis clear, calling them "infidels" and "devil worshippers," but this man was the first ISIS member prosecuted for the crime of genocide against the Yazidi (DW, 2021).

Despite significant evidence of the persecution, displacement, and mass murder of the Rohingya people by the Burmese military that started in 2016, many powerful states, including the US, have been hesitant to label it a genocide. Instead, both the Trump and Biden administrations have called it "ethnic cleansing" (Chishti & Thames, 2021). Ethnic cleansing is not a legal term and does not have an "official" definition per se, but is used colloquially and even in UN resolutions to represent "a purposeful policy designed by one ethnic or religious group to remove by violent and terror-inspiring means the civilian population of another ethnic or religious group from certain geographic areas," as phrased by a UN report on the violations committed in Yugoslavia in the 1990s (UN, 2021a). In simpler terms, all genocide is ethnic cleansing, but not all examples of ethnic cleansing meet the legal standard for genocide.

REFERENCES

Aikins, M., Koettl, C., Hill, E., & Schmitt, E. (2021, September 10). Times investigation: in U.S. drone strike, evidence suggests no ISIS bomb. *The New York Times.* https://www.nytimes.com/2021/09/10/world/asia/us-air-strike-drone-kabul-afghanistan-isis.html.

Amnesty International. (2021). *Detention and imprisonment.* https://www.amnesty.org/en/what-we-do/detention/.

Arms Control Association. (2021a). *Nuclear weapons: who has what at a glance.* Fact Sheets & Briefs. https://www.armscontrol.org/factsheets/Nuclearweapons whohaswhat.

Arms Control Association. (2021b). *Timeline of Syrian chemical weapons activity, 2012–2021.* https://www.armscontrol.org/factsheets/Timeline-of-Syrian-Chemical-Weapons-Activity.

Associated Press (AP). (2017). *Nigerian air force kills more than 100 civilians by accident in strike targeting Boko Haram.* https://www.nbcnews.com/news/world /nigerian-air-force-kills-more-100-civilians-accident-northeastern-strike -n707876.

Beaumont, P. (2014). Witness to a shelling: first-hand account of deadly strike on Gaza port. *The Guardian.* https://www.theguardian.com/world/2014/jul/16 /witness-gaza-shelling-first-hand-account.

Bergen, P., Salyk-Virk, M., & Sterman, D. (2020). World of drones—who has what: countries with armed drones. *New America.* https://www.newamerica.org /international-security/reports/world-drones/.

Bernstein, R. (1988, May 22). U.S. articles on prewar Jews of Germany found wanting. *The New York Times.* https://www.nytimes.com/1988/05/22/us/us-articles -on-prewar-jews-of-germany-found-wanting.html.

Chishti, R., & Thames, K. (2021). *Now is the time to recognize the genocide in Burma.* Atlantic Council. https://www.atlanticcouncil.org/blogs/new-atlanticist/now -is-the-time-to-recognize-the-genocide-in-burma/.

Crawford, N. (2020). Afghanistan's rising civilian death toll due to airstrikes, 2017–2020. https://watson.brown.edu/costsofwar/files/cow/imce/papers/2020 /Rising%20Civilian%20Death%20Toll%20in%20Afghanistan_Costs%20 of%20War_Dec%207%202020.pdf.

Crevecoeur, I., Dias-Meirinho, M. H., Zazzo, A., et al. (2021). New insights on interpersonal violence in the Late Pleistocene based on the Nile valley cemetery of Jebel Sahaba. *Scientific Reports, 11.* https://doi.org/10.1038/s41598-021-89386-y.

Deutsche Welle (DW). (2021, November 30). *German court finds former "IS" member guilty of genocide.* https://www.dw.com/en/german-court-finds-former-is -member-guilty-of-genocide/a-59976226.

Feroz, E. (2021, October 7). After 20 years of drone strikes, it's time to admit they've failed. *MIT Technology Review.* https://www.technologyreview.com /2021/10/07/1036456/opinion-afghanistan-drone-strike-warfare-failed/.

Frischknecht, F. (2003). The history of biological warfare. Human experimentation, modern nightmares and lone madmen in the twentieth century. *EMBO Reports, 4* (Suppl 1), S47–S52. https://doi.org/10.1038/sj.embor.embor849.

The Guardian. (2002, August 27). *Full text of Dick Cheney's speech.* https://www .theguardian.com/world/2002/aug/27/usa.iraq.

The Guardian. (2016, October 15). *Saudi-led coalition admits to bombing Yemen funeral.* https://www.theguardian.com/world/2016/oct/15/saudi-led-coalition -admits-to-bombing-yemen-funeral.

Haar, R. J., Iacopino, V., Ranadive, N., et al. (2017). Death, injury and disability from kinetic impact projectiles in crowd-control settings: a systematic review. *BMJ Open, 7*:e018154. https://doi.org/10.1136/bmjopen-2017-018154.

Hall, R. (Ed.). (1998). *Case studies in strategic bombardment.* Air Force History and Museums Program. https://media.defense.gov/2010/Oct/12/2001330115/-1/-1 /0/AFD-101012-036.pdf.

International Campaign to Abolish Nuclear Weapons (ICAN). (2021). *Hiroshima and Nagasaki bombings.* https://www.icanw.org/hiroshima_and_nagasaki _bombings.

International Campaign to Ban Landmines. (2020). *Landmine monitor 2020.* http://www.the-monitor.org/media/3168934/LM2020.pdf.

International Committee of the Red Cross (ICRC). (2010). *Cluster munitions: what are they and what is the problem?* https://www.icrc.org/en/doc/resources/docu ments/legal-fact-sheet/cluster-munitions-factsheet-230710.htm.

International Committee of the Red Cross (ICRC). (2013). *Chemical and biological weapons.* https://www.icrc.org/en/document/chemical-biological-weapons.

Joshi, H. (2021). *Non-lethal weapons market by technology (chemical, electroshock, mechanical and kinetic, acoustic/light, and others), product type (gases and sprays, grenades, Taser guns, bullets, and others), and end user (law enforcement agencies, military, and citizens): global opportunity analysis and industry forecast, 2021– 2028.* Allied Market Research. https://www.alliedmarketresearch.com/non -lethal-weapons-market.

Karp, A. (2018). *Estimating global military-owned firearms numbers.* Small Arms Survey. https://www.smallarmssurvey.org/sites/default/files/resources/SAS -BP-Military-Firearms-Numbers.pdf.

King, M. (1967). Martin Luther King Jr. on the Vietnam War. *The Atlantic.* https:// www.theatlantic.com/magazine/archive/2018/02/martin-luther-king-jr -vietnam/552521/.

Legacies of War. (2021). *Secret war in Laos.* http://legaciesofwar.org/about-laos /secret-war-laos/.

Mirazón Lahr, M., Rivera, F., Power, R. K., Mounier, A., Copsey, B., Crivellaro, F., Edung, J. E., Maillo Fernandez, J. M., Kiarie, C., Lawrence, J., Leakey, A., Mbua, E., Miller, H., Muigai, A., Mukhongo, D. M., Van Baelen, A., Wood, R., Schwenninger, J. L., Grün, R., Achyuthan, H., . . . Foley, R. A. (2016). Intergroup violence among early Holocene hunter-gatherers of West Turkana, Kenya. *Nature, 529*(7586), 394–398. https://doi.org/10.1038/nature16477.

New Scientist. (n.d.). *The invention of the nuclear bomb.* https://www.newscientist .com/definition/invention-nuclear-bomb/.

Pan, E. (2005). *DEFENSE: non-lethal weapons.* Council on Foreign Relations. https://www.cfr.org/backgrounder/defense-non-lethal-weapons.

Physicians for Human Rights (PHR) (2021). *The aftermath of 9/11: the U.S. torture program in the "War on Terror."* https://phr.org/our-work/resources/twenty -years-of-the-u-s-torture-regime/.

Sands, W. (2021, October 11). My neighbor the tear gas factory. *Mother Jones.* https://www.motherjones.com/anti-racism-police-protest/2021/10/my -neighbor-the-tear-gas-factory/.

Scahill, J. (2015, October 15). The assassination complex. *The Intercept.* https:// theintercept.com/drone-papers/the-assassination-complex/.

Schoch, W., Bigga, G., Böhner, U., Richter, P., & Terberger, T. (2015). New insights on the wooden weapons from the Paleolithic site of Schöningen. *Journal of Human Evolution, 89*, 214–225.

Stockholm International Peace Research Institute (SIPRI). (2020). *Global arms industry: sales by the top 25 companies up 8.5 per cent; big players active in global south.* https://www.sipri.org/media/press-release/2020/global-arms-industry-sales -top-25-companies-85-cent-big-players-active-global-south.

Stojanowski, C. M., Seidel, A. C., Fulginiti, L. C., Johnson, K. M., & Buikstra, J. E. (2016). Contesting the massacre at Nataruk. *Nature, 539*(7630), E8–E10. https:// doi.org/10.1038/nature19778.

Syrian Network for Human Rights (SNHR). (2018). *No less than 13,197 individuals died due to torture, including 167 children and 59 women.* https://sn4hr.org/wp -content/pdf/english/Out_of_sight_en.pdf.

Syrian Network for Human Rights (SNHR). (2021). *In nine years, the Syrian regime has dropped nearly 82,000 barrel bombs, killing 11,087 civilians, including 1,821 children.* https://reliefweb.int/sites/reliefweb.int/files/resources/In_Nine _Years_the_Syrian_Regime_Has_Dropped_Nearly_82%2C000_Barrel_Bombs _Killing_11087_Civilians_Including_1821_Children_en.pdf.

Taylor, A. (2015, April 23). The U.S. keeps killing Americans in drone strikes, mostly by accident. *The Washington Post.* https://www.washingtonpost.com /news/worldviews/wp/2015/04/23/the-u-s-keeps-killing-americans-in -drone-strikes-mostly-by-accident/.

United Nations (UN). (2021a). *Ethnic cleansing.* Office on Genocide Prevention and the Responsibility to Protect. https://www.un.org/en/genocideprevention /ethnic-cleansing.shtml.

United Nations (UN). (2021b). *Genocide.* Office on Genocide Prevention and the Responsibility to Protect. https://www.un.org/en/genocideprevention/geno cide.shtml.

United States Institute of Peace. (2008). *Confronting crimes against humanity.* https://www.usip.org/sites/default/files/Adan/09sg.pdf.

US Army. (2016). *Rifle and carbine training circular (TC) 3-22.9.* https://irp.fas.org/doddir/army/tc3-22-9.pdf.

Von Meding, J. (2017). Agent Orange, exposed: how U.S. chemical warfare in Vietnam unleashed a slow-moving disaster. *The Conversation.* https://theconversation.com/agent-orange-exposed-how-u-s-chemical-warfare-in-vietnam-unleashed-a-slow-moving-disaster-84572.

World Health Organization (WHO). (2002). *World report on violence and health.* https://www.who.int/violence_injury_prevention/violence/world_report/en/full_en.pdf.

World Prison Brief. (2021). *Highest to lowest—prison population total.* https://www.prisonstudies.org/highest-to-lowest/prison-population-total?field_region_taxonomy_tid=All.

Zegart, A. (2020). Cheap fights, credible threats: the future of armed drones and coercion. *Journal of Strategic Studies, 43*(1), 6-46, https://doi.org/10.1080/01402390.2018.1439747.

CHAPTER 4

INTERPERSONAL AND SELF-DIRECTED VIOLENCE

Never, for any reason on earth, could you wish for an increase of
pain. Of pain you could only wish for one thing: that it should stop.
Nothing in the world was so bad as physical pain. In the face of pain
there are no heroes, no heroes, he thought over and over as he
writhed on the floor, clutching uselessly at his disabled left arm.

—GEORGE ORWELL, *1984* (1949)

Fed through the tube that sticks in me
Just like a wartime novelty
Tied to machines that make me be
Cut this life off from me.

—METALLICA, "One" (1989)

AS THE GUN VIOLENCE epidemic in the United States has accelerated
in recent decades, research increasingly suggests that, in many cases of
mass shootings or terrorism, there is a trail of abuse and violence leading up to the event. Adam Lanza, the man who killed 20 children and six
adults at Sandy Hook Elementary School in 2012, first killed his mother
that morning. The perpetrator of the mass school shooting in Uvalde,

Texas, in 2022, Salvador Ramos, shot his grandmother in the face before he made his way to Robb Elementary School and killed 19 children and two teachers. The wife of Omar Mateen, the man who killed 49 people in the Pulse nightclub shooting in 2016, claimed that during their entire marriage, he physically, verbally, and sexually assaulted her; his ex-wife had left him after four months for the same reasons.

Stephen Paddock, who perpetrated what remains the deadliest mass shooting by an individual in the history of the United States when he killed 60 people in Las Vegas, had a history of verbally abusing his girlfriend in public, as well as a cache of hundreds of images of child pornography on his computer. Micah Johnson, a former Army reservist who killed five police officers and injured several more in Dallas in 2016, was discharged from a tour of Afghanistan for stalking and harassing a fellow service member. His former bunkmate reportedly wrote on Facebook, "We all knew he was a pervert cuz [sic] he got caught stealing girls' panties but murdering cops is a different story" (Stepansky & Dillon, 2016).

Surely not every individual who commits individual acts of violence or harassment will perpetrate an act of mass violence, but evidence suggests that most who commit an act of mass violence will have a record of interpersonal violence, usually against women (we'll explore the significant gender dimensions of violence later). A 2021 study found that, between 2014 and 2019, 60% of mass shooting incidents involved a shooter with a history of domestic violence, and that shootings related to domestic violence had a higher case fatality rate than others (Geller, Booty, & Crifasi, 2021).

It is always difficult, of course, to extrapolate these incidents to behaviors in environments of armed conflict; for example, Bashar al-Assad, ultimately responsible for the deaths, disappearance, torture, and displacement of millions of Syrians, had a reputation as a "mild-mannered," "shy," even "geeky" ophthalmologist, who avoided military service and was not his father's first choice for successor. However, they do provide evidence to disabuse us of the notion that mass violence is not preventable or predictable. Not only can interpersonal violence lead to collective violence, but the environment of armed conflict can provide fertile ground for greater interpersonal violence.

Interpersonal violence can be physical, psychological, or sexual in nature, perpetrated by or against a single individual or a small group. There are two forms of interpersonal violence: family or partner violence (such as intimate partner abuse, elder abuse, or child abuse) and community violence, which occurs between people who are not part of the same household but otherwise interact within a community setting. This may include bullying, rape, or assault (Mercy et al., 2017). Interpersonal violence exists in every setting, among every race and ethnicity, and across all geographies and demographics; which makes it difficult to connect the dots between the violence that happens in the home, in the workplace, or at school, with the mass violence that defines armed conflict.

This can become even more puzzling when considering self-directed violence, which the CDC defines as anything a person does intentionally that can cause self-injury, including suicide and self-mutilation (e.g., cutting). This type of violence happens everywhere; it's not limited to the war environment. But while the literature does suggest increases in all types of violence during and after conflict, these are also the consequences of an overly militarized society, where violence or the threats of violence are viewed as a posture of strength rather than weakness.

Although the violence of war is primarily focused on the population-level, its effects are not limited to this level. The violence and trauma inherent in the war environment trickles down to the interpersonal and individual levels, causing injury and death, whose connection to the conflict often goes unrecognized. This prevents us from gauging the full ramifications of how armed conflict harms civilians, especially those who do not directly experience battle-related injury from weapons.

Interpersonal violence is a significant global issue: of the 4.4 million injury-related deaths per year, only 1 in 61 directly result from war or conflict, yet 1 in 10 are from homicide and 1 in 6 are due to suicide. For children and young adults aged 5–29, homicide and suicide are two of the top five causes of death globally (WHO, 2021b). Many of these deaths occur in countries that are not conflict-affected or even considered fragile by the World Bank standard. In fact, the region of the Americas has the highest interpersonal violence rate in the world, and is the only region where this ranks as a top 10 cause of death (WHO, 2019).

Deaths by suicide are not necessarily intuitively distributed, either. The region with the highest suicide rate is the continent of Africa, followed by Europe. The Eastern Mediterranean, the region with the most conflicts, ranks lowest, while the Americas is the only region where the rate is increasing (WHO, 2021c). How can this possibly fit in with war?

INTERPERSONAL VIOLENCE

Evidence of what we assume to be interpersonal violence significantly predates the first purported evidence of collective violence. It can be difficult to parse out causes of death thousands—let alone hundreds of thousands—of years after the fact: was that cranial damage evidence of abuse or murder, or was it experienced postmortem due to centuries of pressure from rocks? If it was violence, was it an animal? Was it a hunting accident? While it is nearly impossible to determine circumstances or motives from the condition of fossilized remains, today's archeologists have ways of telling whether injuries were intentional or not, and whether they occurred before or after death.

In 2015, scientists analyzed evidence from one of the first documented potential murder victims. Painstaking examination found that the victim, who lived approximately 430,000 years ago, was likely killed by being struck in the head twice with the same object (Sala et al., 2015). In fact, more so than any form of documentation or written record, analysis of human remains shows that interpersonal violence, especially by and towards men, has been prevalent throughout history. A comprehensive review of the bioarcheological evidence of violence concluded, "As far as we know, there are no forms of social organization, modes of production, or environmental settings that remain free from interpersonal violence for long" (Walker, 2001).

All this early evidence of violence—doesn't it mean that violence is inherently human and impossible to stop? Current figures certainly support that perspective. The WHO estimates that 1 in 3 women in the world has been subjected to physical or sexual violence in their lifetime; 1 billion children have experienced physical, sexual, or emotional violence in the past year; and about 1 in 6 people aged 60 or older has experienced elder abuse. Unlike collective violence, there is seldom a political motive for interpersonal violence, with the notable exceptions of incidents of violence driven by politically induced bigotry—such as persecution of sexual, religious, or ethnic minorities—and violence against political figures.

The seemingly inevitable nature of violence of all kinds, at all levels, appears intractable. Yet there are many well-established risk factors for interpersonal violence, including poverty and economic inequality, weak economic and social safety nets, gender inequality, substance use and abuse, and cultural norms of accepting violence (Phinney & de Hovre, 2003). In fact, many of these same dynamics are considered risk factors for collective violence and armed conflict. Additional individual-level risk factors include untreated mental health ailments—such as antisocial personality disorder, schizophrenia, and non-schizophrenic psychotic disorders—and, significantly, witnessing or experiencing violence in childhood (Fazel, Smith, Chang, & Geddes, 2018).

War, of course, provides the perfect mix of economic insecurity, lack of health care access (including for mental health), and other factors that exacerbate violence. After decades of steady decline, the homicide rate in the United States more than doubled during the Vietnam War, as did the homicide rate in Italy after World War II. In fact, domestic homicide rates have been shown to increase after war in every circumstance: whether the war was fought at home or abroad; whether or not the state was victorious; whatever the condition of the postwar economy; and in all demographics. This indicates that it's not societal disorganization, economic disruption, or any other commonly considered factor affecting such numbers: it is simply the legitimation of violence. The authors of a seminal study that reported these findings concluded, "Wars provide concrete evidence that homicide, under some conditions, is acceptable in the eyes of a nation's leaders. The wartime reversal of the customary peacetime prohibition against killing may somehow influence the threshold for using homicide as a means of settling conflict in everyday life" (Archer & Gartner, 1976).

Later studies offered additional explanations for violence rates. These include exposure to violence in video games and movies; and, in the case of countries like the United States (where active conflict is almost never experienced), the official sanction of corporal punishment, the death penalty, permissive gun laws, mass incarceration, and extrajudicial police shootings, all of which help to legitimize violence in civilian populations (Stamatel & Romans, 2018). And it's not just crime. Research shows that when police forces are militarized—in many cases, quite literally given surplus military weapons and vehicles—civilians are more likely to be killed by police (Delehanty, Mewhirter, Welch, & Wilks, 2017).

DOMESTIC VIOLENCE

Domestic and family violence is the most well-addressed form of interpersonal violence in the conflict literature. Across conflict environments, and even in post-conflict settings, this type of violence increases. Much of this violence is perpetuated by men against women and children. As one study hypothesizes, "When hyper-masculinized and traumatized male combatants leave the battlefield, often, for a myriad of reasons, their homes become new stages for violence" (Bradley, 2018). Indeed, in humanitarian settings, it's not just substance use, socioeconomic status, mental health, or lack of social support that is associated with increased violence in the home—it's also exposure to the conflict environment (Rubenstein, Lu, MacFarlane, & Stark, 2020).

According to a study from Liberia, living in an area that experienced conflict fatalities increased the risk of intimate partner violence (IPV) by 60%, and increased the risk of injury from IPV within the previous year by 50% (Kelly, Colantuoni, Robinson, & Decker, 2021). We'll discuss the gendered aspects of violence, specifically violence against women, in more detail in a later chapter; but for now, it is important to note that living in the war environment adds to the risk of violence for women in the home, including for spouses of men in the armed forces. Since 2015, more than 100,000 incidents of domestic abuse have been reported to the US military. Many of these cases are ignored or closed quickly.

One military spouse, who reported her husband's abuse of her to the Army while she and her husband were deployed in South Korea, spoke with CBS News about her story. The military, she said, found cause to charge her husband. The punishment? A letter of reprimand from his commander, which was expunged from his record once he left the deployment. As she told the reporter, "The soldier is an asset. They need him. They have spent a lot of money to train him to do his job. And who am I?" (O'Donnell et al., 2021).

VIOLENCE AGAINST CHILDREN

With regard to children, findings are a bit more nuanced. About 426 million children lived in a conflict zone in 2019 (40% in the Middle East alone), while 1.6 billion lived in a country somehow affected by conflict (Østby, Rustad, & Tollefsen, 2020). According to the UN, a child dies every five minutes due to violence. For a child in the war environment, having a parent who exhibits warmth and sensitivity can be highly protective against the trauma of their experience. Of course, parenting in any environment is stressful, and parenting in the war environment is an especially significant stressor. Some parents mishandle these pressures by taking out their stress and anxiety on their child, either through abuse or neglect.

Conversely, parents may worry excessively about their child, and be overly restrictive and controlling. The parent's response may depend on the type of conflict exposure. For example, in highly insecure settings, parents may be more likely to exhibit harshness and hostility to their children, while in settings that are merely under threat, parents may be more warm, but also overprotective (Eltanamly, Leijten, Jak, & Overbeek, 2019).

The personal experiences of the parents are the surest predictors of child abuse or neglect. Even in the stressful war environment, parents of both genders who have been abused as children are more likely to be aggressive toward their own, as are women who have been victimized by their intimate partner, and men who experience symptoms of PTSD or report high alcohol use (Saile, Ertl, Neuner, & Catani, 2014). It's difficult to get an accurate read on rates of child abuse in even the wealthiest and most politically stable countries, let alone in the war environment. But war is likely to increase the factors that put children at a higher risk of abuse by the adults in their lives; and as these children are victimized, they are more likely, as adults, to victimize their own children.

On top of the increased risk of violence in the home, in extremely fragile settings, children as young as eight years old may even be recruited and used as soldiers, cooks, messengers, scouts, and, most often in the case of young girls, sex slaves for militants. UNICEF estimates that, from 2005 to 2020, at least 93,000 children were used as what are generally called "child soldiers" in various conflicts around the world. These children may be exploited for dangerous labor (including producing bombs), coerced to use drugs, and, of course, injured and abused physically, or damaged psychologically, by being forced to inflict or witness violence against others (2021). In 2000, the Optional Protocol to the Convention on the Rights of the Child on the Involvement of Children in Armed Conflict was adopted by the UN General Assembly, prohibiting the use of children younger than 18 in hostilities. Recruiting children under the age of 15 is also considered a war crime under international humanitarian law, but the practice continues in countries like Afghanistan, Myanmar, Somalia, Sudan, South Sudan, and Yemen (UN, 2021).

Aside from the children of families living in conflict, children of members of the armed forces also suffer an increased risk of domestic violence, even when far removed from the conflict itself. Data on this topic, while relevant to every country with a military, is especially focused on the United States, where there are nearly two million children in military families. After the United States escalated the wars in Iraq and Afghanistan in 2002, rates of child mistreatment in military families surged as well, especially when the soldier was on combat-related deployment. Child mistreatment rates are 42% higher during the deployment than non-deployment (Sogomonyan & Cooper, 2010). Children may be abused or neglected by the non-deployed family member, who may be experiencing increased stress due to being alone for long periods of time; or abused by the returning military family member, who may be experiencing PTSD, other mental ailments, or an undetected traumatic brain injury that changes behavior and increases aggression.

As with intimate partner violence, the insular nature of the military seems to further enable child abusers to avoid accountability. In 2016, President Barack Obama signed "Talia's Law," after five-year-old Talia Williams was tortured and beaten to death by her active-duty Army father on a military base in Hawaii. Multiple individuals, including military police, doctors, and employees at the on-base childcare facility, failed to report obvious signs of abuse. The law would require anyone employed by the Defense Department to report suspected child abuse on bases to state agencies, as well as up the military chain of command (Gerber, 2016). That said, since the military has historically responded poorly to charges of domestic violence or sexual assault in their ranks, it seems clear that incidents of child abuse and related fatalities are underreported.

Research on this topic, unfortunately, is exceedingly sparse; although one study found that from 2004 to 2007, of 5,945 confirmed cases of mistreatment of children in Army families, only 20% had a formal report in the Army Family Advocacy Program system (Wood et al., 2017). "There's a real reluctance to address child-abuse fatalities in the military because it's a career ender for soldiers," according to the head of the National Center for the Review and Prevention of Child Deaths (Cloud, 2016).

ELDER ABUSE

Elder abuse is among the least studied forms of interpersonal violence, but intermittent reports suggest that it is not atypical, affecting at least 15% of elderly adults worldwide (at least 141 million people). Data is especially sparse from low- and middle-income countries, where most conflicts are waged (Yon, Mikton, Gassoumis, & Wilber, 2017). It can come in the form of physical, sexual, and psychological abuse, neglect, and financial exploitation. Those with dementia or Alzheimer's disease are at especially high risks of being abused (Dong, 2015), as are elderly persons in unsupervised settings and those in family units disrupted by widowhood, divorce, or separation (Vida, Monks, & Des Rosiers, 2002). There are few if any studies assessing elder abuse in the war setting, but it seems to make sense that in an environment where mentally impaired elderly adults cannot receive adequate treatment, families are facing high caregiving burdens, and many families are disrupted by trauma and loss, this form of interpersonal abuse may follow. Further, elders in war environments are often entirely dependent on their families and are the most affected by loss of social support. In Yemen, for example, 95% of elderly adults have no access to income, less than 3% can afford their own medications, and more than half cannot access health care if needed (HelpAge International, 2021). In these conditions of extreme dependence, the potential for abuse and neglect is high.

As meager as the data is about elder abuse in the war zone, data from veteran populations is just as scarce. The US Department of Veterans Affairs, or VA, estimates that in 2018, there were more than 11 million veterans above the age of 60, more than half of the approximately 20 million total living veterans (2021). However, the VA has engaged in little research of abuse of elderly veterans, despite the significant risk factors faced by the aging veteran population. These include a higher likelihood of PTSD; poor physical health (at least two or more chronic medical conditions) and mental health (the VA estimates that 18–28% of veterans had dementia in 2014); and a higher propensity for social isolation and loneliness (Makaroun, Taylor, & Rosen, 2018).

The lack of insightful investigation of elder abuse is hardly limited to war and military contexts—being an oversight of public health in general—but the absence of meaningful inquiry by the VA, one of the largest health care providers in the country, is stark, considering the "thank you for your service" culture that is so pervasive in the United States.

SELF-DIRECTED VIOLENCE

September 11, 2001, was unquestionably a pivotal day in modern history—a rare violent attack by a foreign entity on American soil, killing thousands of people. However, aside from what happened on the day itself, the significance of that day and the events that followed have become even clearer in the subsequent decades. The United States and its allies began military offensives on multiple fronts, starting with wars in Iraq and Afghanistan that were soon used to justify operations throughout the Middle East and Africa. As a result, more was asked of US service members than in any previous conflict, including multiple long deployments, many to live combat zones. Almost half of post-9/11 veterans reported emotionally traumatic or distressing experiences—double the rate of pre-9/11 veterans—and 45% said the military did not adequately prepare them for the transition back to civilian life, compared to only 21% of pre-9/11 veterans (Parker, Igielnik, Barroso, & Cilluffo, 2019).

Yet it is still shocking to learn that more American active-duty personnel and veterans of the post-9/11 wars died by suicide than died in combat—in fact, more than four times as many (30,000 suicides vs. 7,000 killed in action). A report from the Costs of War project suggests that such factors as military culture, high exposure to trauma and stress, easy access to guns, difficulty reintegrating into civilian life, the long length of wars, heightened risk of traumatic brain injury, and the public's uninterest in the ongoing wars all contributed to this significant disparity (Suitt, 2021). While most available research is focused on the US Armed Forces, research from other countries indicates that suicide is a health concern in other armed forces as well, including in France (Desjeux, Labarère, Galoisy-Guibal, & Ecochard, 2004) and Germany (Helms, Wertenauer, Spaniol, Zimmermann, & Willmund, 2021).

When we consider self-directed violence, suicide generally comes to mind. According to the Global Burden of Disease study, suicide is one of the leading causes of death globally. About 800,000 people die by suicide each year—double the amount that die from homicide, and more than six times as many as from conflict (Roth et al., 2018). As the WHO notes, for every reported suicide there are numerous unreported suicide attempts, and many deaths by suicide are not accurately reported at all, due either to inadequate data or cultural and religious stigmas. More than three-quarters of suicides (77%) occur in low- and middle-income countries, and primary methods include hanging, firearms, and self-poisoning (2021a, 2021c).

Suicide, perhaps more so than other forms of violence, is considered contagious, in that "suicide clusters" can occur when exposures to suicide, especially in the peer group or with the widely reported suicide of a celebrity, increase. A review of this phenomenon notes that the infectious disease model can easily be applied to suicide contagion, and that "a suicide cluster can be seen as behaving like an epidemic" (Haw, Hawton, Niedzwiedz, & Platt, 2013).

Further, in a militarized society like the United States, guns are easily accessible, and households with more guns report higher rates of suicide by gun. Guns are, by far, the most commonly used means of suicide in the United States, and the most likely to result in death. This is not to say that gun ownership leads to suicide, but an individual with suicidal ideation who is able to access a gun may be more likely to reach for it in an impulsive moment (RAND, 2018).

Contrary to what conventional wisdom might tell us about suicide among civilians in the war environment, much of the historical data we have suggests that suicide actually decreases during war. The initial hypothesis was that war provides a common enemy and increases bonding and social ties within societies. Later work found that, when controlling for unemployment, war did not meaningfully influence suicide rates, and that the economic effects of conflict were more impactful on suicide rates than war itself (Lester & Yang, 1991). Much of these works focused on the American population or populations during interstate wars, but later research on non-US populations and civil wars showed the same pattern.

In Sri Lanka, for example, suicide decreased by 43% to 52% during the civil war in the 1980s and 1990s (Aida, 2020). The same trend was found in Croatia, where suicide rates decreased in areas affected by war, although methods of suicide differed. Non-conflict-affected areas reported more suicides from hangings, whereas firearms and explosives were more frequently used in affected areas (Grubisić-Ilić, Kozarić-Kovacić, Grubisić, & Kovacić, 2002). Indeed, World Bank data shows that suicide rates in fragile and conflict-affected countries are lower than the world average by almost half (2019).

That said, human resilience may only go so far. Evidence from Nazi and Soviet concentration camps show suicide rates up to 30 times higher than the general population's, although there is evidence that Nazi authorities would use suicide as a cover for murders they committed. Other self-destructive behaviors, like self-mutilation, were also widely reported (López-Muñoz & Cuerda-Galindo, 2016). Initial evidence from

Uyghurs who had been held in detention camps suggests high suicidal ideation (Maizland, 2021), and Rohingya refugees also reported high suicidal ideation, with some saying to counsellors that they already had ropes and pesticides ready at their home (Tay et al., 2019). Many threatened suicide if forced to repatriate to Myanmar, knowing what might await them upon their return (UN, 2018).

In 2020, the UN expressed concern over increasing suicide rates among young adults in the Gaza Strip, citing the ongoing blockade, poor living conditions, high youth unemployment (70%), high poverty (50%), and, significantly, lack of hope. As one physician noted, "I've worked in other countries such as Cambodia but there was a political process and international support that gave hope. Here we just keep people breathing."

While rigorous work on this topic is lacking, these examples indicate some nuance in these non-intuitive numbers. Situations in which civilians feel hopeless, are economically desperate, or are held in particularly inhumane conditions may also indicate a higher likelihood of suicide. A friend of a young man who died by suicide in the Gaza Strip wrote, "Increasingly lonely, broke, and constantly harassed, Suleiman found a way out of the Gaza cage. But it was to his grave" (Shehada, 2020).

There are other distinctions to be found regarding suicide and war that can help tease out some of the main areas of concern. A study from Nepal found that former child soldiers reported suicidal ideation, plans, and attempts at double the rates of their civilian counterparts, especially among females who had experienced sexual violence (Bhardwaj et al., 2018). And, disturbingly, children are often used in suicide bombings, which are a unique and dangerous combination of interpersonal and self-directed violence. Suicide bombings have been used for more than 130 years in over 40 countries and territories; it is estimated that, over that time span, approximately 13,500 suicide attacks have killed at least 50,000 people.

The term "suicide bomber" is slightly misleading, because some of the perpetrators, especially children and people with mental disabilities, may be forced or manipulated into partaking in the bombing. We are all familiar with the Japanese kamikaze pilots of World War II, but after that, suicide bombings were not widely used until the 1980s. They've since had a resurgence, mostly throughout the Middle East and Asia, in attacks by militant groups in Lebanon, Sri Lanka, the occupied Palestinian territories, Pakistan, Russia, Iraq, Chad, Cameroon, Nigeria, Afghanistan, etc. (Overton, 2020).

Perhaps the most infamous examples of suicide terrorism, however, were the attacks on the United States on September 11, 2001. While many of these attackers have been dismissed merely as religious or political fanatics, evidence suggests that those who willfully consent to sacrifice themselves in suicide attacks are, like many others who contemplate suicide, depressed, suffering from PTSD, or overwhelmed with feelings of hopelessness. Many suicide attackers, according to research, previously attempted suicide in one way or another, prior to their attempted or completed attack (Lankford, 2015b).

Interestingly, there has been an increase in research on the characteristics of mass shooters in the United States, including school shooters, that suggest that these individuals are more likely to resemble those who die by suicide as opposed to other types of homicidal offenders, as many intend to take their own lives once they have committed the shooting or once authorities make it to the scene to end the shooting (Lankford, Silver, & Cox, 2021). They may also purposefully taunt or threaten police who arrive at the scene to orchestrate what is colloquially called "suicide by cop." While the United States, a country not experiencing active warfare on its own territory, is the country with the most mass shootings, the connections between these types of crimes and terrorism—including the targeting of what are often complete strangers in a public setting—make it important to understand the link between perpetration of mass violence of all kinds and suicidal ideation (Lankford, 2015a).

REFERENCES

Aida, T. (2020). Revisiting suicide rate during wartime: evidence from the Sri Lankan civil war. *PLoS ONE, 15*(10): e0240487.

Archer, D., & Gartner, R. (1976). Violent acts and violent times: a comparative approach to postwar homicide rates. *American Sociological Review, 41*(6), 937–963.

Bhardwaj, A., Bourey, C., Rai, S., Adhikari, R., Worthman, C., & Kohrt, B. (2018). Interpersonal violence and suicidality among former child soldiers and war-exposed civilian children in Nepal. *Global Mental Health, 5*, E9. doi:10.1017/gmh.2017.31.

Bradley, S. (2018). Domestic and family violence in post-conflict communities. *Health and Human Rights, 20*(2), 123–136.

Cloud, D. (2016, December 29). Child abuse in the military is another tragic repercussion of years of war. *The Seattle Times*. https://www.seattletimes.com/nation-world/child-abuse-in-the-military-is-another-tragic-repercussion-of-years-of-war/.

Delehanty, C., Mewhirter, J., Welch, R., & Wilks, J. (2017). Militarization and police violence: the case of the 1033 program. *Research & Politics, 4*(2), 1-7.

Desjeux, G., Labarère, J., Galoisy-Guibal, L., & Ecochard, R. (2004). Suicide in the French Armed Forces. *European Journal of Epidemiology, 19*(9), 823–829. http://www.jstor.org/stable/3582593.

Dong, X. (2015). Elder abuse: systematic review and implications for practice. *Journal of the American Geriatric Society, 63*(6), 1214–1238.

Eltanamly, H., Leijten, P., Jak, S., & Overbeek, G. (2021). Parenting in times of war: a meta-analysis and qualitative synthesis of war exposure, parenting, and child adjustment. *Trauma, Violence, & Abuse, 22*(1), 147–160. https://doi.org/10.1177/1524838019833001.

Fazel, S., Smith, N., Chang, Z., & Geddes, J. (2018). Risk factors for interpersonal violence: an umbrella review of meta-analyses. *The British Journal of Psychiatry, 213*, 609–614.

Geller, L., Booty, M., & Crifasi, C. (2021). The role of domestic violence in fatal mass shootings in the United States, 2014–2019. *Injury Epidemiology, 8*(38). https://doi.org/10.1186/s40621-021-00330-0.

Gerber, D. (2016, February 9). Congress moves to confront military child abuse with Talia's Law. *Military Times*. https://www.militarytimes.com/spouse/2016/02/10/congress-moves-to-confront-military-child-abuse-with-talia-s-law/.

Grubisić-Ilić, M., Kozarić-Kovacić, D., Grubisić, F., & Kovacić, Z. (2002). Epidemiological study of suicide in the Republic of Croatia—comparison of war and post-war periods and areas directly and indirectly affected by war. *European Psychiatry: The Journal of the Association of European Psychiatrists, 17*(5), 259–264. https://doi.org/10.1016/s0924-9338(02)00679-x.

Haw, C., Hawton, K., Niedzwiedz, C., & Platt, S. (2013). Suicide clusters: a review of risk factors and mechanisms. *Suicide and Life-Threatening Behavior, 43*(1), 97–108.

Helms, C., Wertenauer, F., Spaniol, K. U., Zimmermann, P. L., & Willmund, G. D. (2021). Suicidal behavior in German military service members: an analysis of attempted and completed suicides between 2010 and 2016. *PloS ONE, 16*(8), e0256104. https://doi.org/10.1371/journal.pone.0256104.

HelpAge International. (2021). *Older people's lives at risk as war in Yemen leaves them struggling for food, income and medication.* https://www.helpage.org/newsroom /press-room/press-releases/older-peoples-lives-at-risk-as-war-in-yemen -leaves-them-struggling-for-food-income-and-medication/.

Jewkes, R., Jama-Shai, N., & Sikweyiya, Y. (2017). Enduring impact of conflict on mental health and gender-based violence perpetration in Bougainville, Papua New Guinea: a cross-sectional study. *PLoS ONE, 12*(10): e0186062. https://doi .org/10.1371/journal.pone.0186062.

Kelly, J., Colantuoni, E., Robinson, C., & Decker, M. (2021). How armed conflict is associated with more severe violence in the home. *Health and Human Rights Journal, 23*(1), 75–89.

Lankford, A. (2015a). Mass shooters in the USA, 1966–2010: differences between attackers who live and die. *Justice Quarterly, 32*(2), 360–379, https://doi.org/10 .1080/07418825.2013.806675.

Lankford, A. (2015b). What you don't understand about suicide attacks. *Scientific American.* https://www.scientificamerican.com/article/what-you-don-t-under stand-about-suicide-attacks/.

Lankford, A., Silver, J., & Cox, J. (2021). An epidemiological analysis of public mass shooters and active shooters: quantifying key differences between perpetrators and the general population, homicide offenders, and people who die by suicide. *Journal of Threat Assessment and Management, 8*(4), 125–144.

Lester, D., & Yang, B. (1991). The influence of war on suicide rates. *The Journal of Social Psychology, 132*(1), 135-137.

López-Muñoz, F., & Cuerda-Galindo, E. (2016). Suicide in inmates in Nazi and Soviet concentration camps: historical overview and critique. *Frontiers in Psy-chiatry, 7*, 88. https://doi.org/10.3389/fpsyt.2016.00088.

Maizland, L. (2021). *China's repression of Uyghurs in Xinjiang.* Council on Foreign Relations. https://www.cfr.org/backgrounder/chinas-repression-uyghurs-xin jiang.

Makaroun, L., Taylor, L., & Rosen, T. (2018). Veterans experiencing elder abuse: improving care for a high-risk population about which little is known. *Journal of the American Geriatrics Society, 66*(2), 389-393.

Mercy, J. A., Hillis, S. D., Butchart, A., et al. (2017). Interpersonal violence: global impact and paths to prevention. In C. N. Mock, R. Nugent, O. Kobusingye et al. (Eds.). *Injury prevention and environmental health* (3rd ed., Chapter 5). Washington, DC: International Bank for Reconstruction and Development; The World Bank.

O'Donnell, N., Steve, K., Tepper, L., Verdugo, A., & Yilek, C. (2021). "It was severe betrayal": military has failed to address domestic violence, survivors say. *CBS News*. https://www.cbsnews.com/news/military-domestic-violence-survivors -investigation-norah-odonnell-cbs-news/.

Østby, G., Rustad, S., & Tollefsen, A. (2020). *Children affected by armed conflict, 1990–2019*. Peace Research Institute Oslo. https://www.prio.org/publications /12527.

Overton, I. (2020). *A short history of suicide bombing*. Action on Armed Violence. https://aoav.org.uk/2020/a-short-history-of-suicide-bombings/.

Parker, K., Igielnik, R., Barroso, A., & Cilluffo, A. (2019). *The American veteran experience and the post 9/11 generation*. Pew Research Center. https://www.pewre search.org/social-trends/2019/09/10/the-american-veteran-experience-and -the-post-9-11-generation/.

Phinney, A., & de Hovre, S. (2003). Integrating human rights and public health to prevent interpersonal violence. *Health and Human Rights, 6*(2), 65–87.

RAND. (2018). *The relationship between firearm availability and suicide*. RAND Corporation. https://www.rand.org/research/gun-policy/analysis/essays/firearm -availability-suicide.html.

Roth, G. A., Abate, D., Abate, K. H., Abay, S. M., Abbafati, C., Abbasi, N., . . . & Abdollahpour, I. (2018). Global, regional, and national age-sex-specific mortality for 282 causes of death in 195 countries and territories, 1980–2017: a systematic analysis for the Global Burden of Disease Study 2017. *The Lancet, 392*(10159), 1736–1788.

Rubenstein, B., Lu, L., MacFarlane, M., & Stark, L. (2020). Predictors of interpersonal violence in the household in humanitarian settings: a systematic review. *Trauma, Violence & Abuse, 21*(1) 31–44.

Saile, R., Ertl, V., Neuner, F., & Catani, C. (2014). Does war contribute to family violence against children? Findings from a two-generational multi-informant study in Northern Uganda. *Child Abuse & Neglect, 38*(1), 135–146.

Sala, N., Arsuaga, J. L., Pantoja-Pérez, A., Pablos, A., Martínez, I., et al. (2015). Lethal interpersonal violence in the Middle Pleistocene. *PLoS ONE 10*(5): e0126589. https://doi.org/10.1371/journal.pone.0126589.

Shehada, M. (2020, June 15). When hope dies: why so many young Palestinians in Gaza are committing suicide. *Haaretz.* https://www.haaretz.com/middle -east-news/.premium-when-hope-died-why-so-many-young-palestinians-in -gaza-are-committing-suicide-1.8995929.

Sogomonyan, F., & Cooper, J. (2010). *Trauma faced by children of military families.* National Center for Children in Poverty. https://www.nccp.org/wp-content /uploads/2010/05/text_938.pdf.

Stamatel, J. P., & Romans, S. H. (2018). The effects of wars on postwar homicide rates: a replication and extension of Archer and Gartner's classic study. *Journal of Contemporary Criminal Justice, 34*(3), 287–311.

Stepansky, J., & Dillon, N. (2016). Dallas cop shooter Micah Johnson was booted from Afghanistan amid sexual harassment accusations. *New York Daily News.* https://www.nydailynews.com/news/national/dallas-shooter-accused -sexual-harassment-army-tour-article-1.2705323.

Suitt, T. (2021). *High suicide rates among United States service members and veterans of the post-9/11 wars* (Working paper). https://watson.brown.edu/costsofwar /files/cow/imce/papers/2021/Suitt_Suicides_Costs%20of%20War_June%20 21%202021.pdf.

Tay, A., Riley, A., Islam, R., Welton-Mitchell, C., Duchesne, B., Water, V., Varner, A., Moussa, B., Mahmudul Alam, N., Elshazly, M., Silove, D., & Ventevogel, P. (2019). The culture, mental health and psychosocial wellbeing of Rohingya refugees: a systematic review. *Epidemiology and Psychiatric Sciences, 28*(5), 489–494.

United Nations (UN). (2018). *Bachelet: returning Rohingya refugees to Myanmar would place them at serious risk of human rights violations.* https://www.ohchr .org/en/press-releases/2018/11/bachelet-returning-rohingya-refugees -myanmar-would-place-them-serious-risk.

United Nations (UN). (2021). *Child recruitment and use.* Office of the Special Representative of the Secretary-General for Children and Armed Conflict. https:// childrenandarmedconflict.un.org/six-grave-violations/child-soldiers/.

UNICEF. (2021). *Children recruited by armed forces and armed groups.* https://www .unicef.org/protection/children-recruited-by-armed-forces.

UN OCHA. (2020). *Deterioration in the mental health situation in the Gaza Strip.* https://www.ochaopt.org/content/deterioration-mental-health-situation -gaza-strip.

Veterans Affairs (VA). (2021). *Population tables—age/gender.* https://www.va.gov /vetdata/veteran_population.asp.

Vida, S., Monks, R., & Des Rosiers, P. (2002). Prevalence and correlates of elder abuse and neglect in a geriatric psychiatry service. *Canadian Journal of Psychiatry, 47*, 459–467.

Walker, P. (2001). A bioarchaeological perspective on the history of violence. *Annual Review of Anthropology, 30*, 573–596.

Wood, J., Griffis, H., Taylor, C., Strane, D., Harb, G., Mi, L., Song, L., Lynch, K., & Rubin, D. (2017). Under-ascertainment from health care settings of child abuse events among children of soldiers by the U.S. Army Family Advocacy Program. *Child Abuse & Neglect, 63*, 202–210.

World Bank. (2019). *Suicide mortality rate (per 100,000 population)—fragile and conflict affected situations.* https://data.worldbank.org/indicator/SH.STA.SUIC .P5?locations=F1-1W.

World Health Organization (WHO). (2019). *Leading causes of death and disability 2000-2019: A visual summary.* https://www.who.int/data/stories/leading -causes-of-death-and-disability-2000-2019-a-visual-summary.

World Health Organization (WHO). (2021a). *Suicide.* https://www.who.int/news -room/fact-sheets/detail/suicide.

World Health Organization (WHO). (2021b). *Injuries and violence.* https://www .who.int/news-room/fact-sheets/detail/injuries-and-violence.

World Health Organization (WHO). (2021c). *Suicide worldwide in 2019.* https:// www.who.int/publications/i/item/9789240026643.

Yon, Y., Mikton, C. R., Gassoumis, Z. D., & Wilber, K. H. (2017). Elder abuse prevalence in community settings: a systematic review and meta-analysis. *The Lancet: Global Health, 5*(2), e147–e156. https://doi.org/10.1016/S2214-109X(17)30006-2.

CHAPTER 5

STRUCTURAL VIOLENCE IN WAR

For the master's tools will never dismantle the master's house. They may allow us to temporarily beat him at his own game, but they will never enable us to bring about genuine change.

—AUDRE LORDE,
comments at "The Personal and the Political" panel (1979)

I have grown weary of telling myself lies
that I might one day begin to believe. We are not all left
standing after the war has ended. Some of us have
become ghosts by the time the dust has settled.

—CLINT SMITH,
"When people say, 'we have made it through worse before'" (2019)

MY UNCLE, THE ONE REFERENCED in the introduction to this book, is among the most mild-mannered men I've ever met. Everyone likes him; he's one of those men of a certain age that you respect and admire. He has an intangible aura of competence and understanding; he's well-read, he's traveled the world, he's taught English to thousands of students. This is not a violent man. This is a man who has quietly built a life over the better part of a century in an impossible place. He's never been in the military, and he's not antagonistic with the soldiers he's been forced to interact with almost every day of his life. When there is direct violence in his town, he *tsks* (much like his sister, my mother, does) and raises his eyebrows, as if to say, *what can you do.* Yet his life, and the lives of his parents, siblings, children, and now, grandchildren, has been dictated by violence—the same kind of violence that almost prevented him from receiving life-saving medical care. Not just individual acts of oppression, but *systems* of oppression, many considered legal by the entities that practice them.

Structural violence is often hard to see, and that's by design. Many systems of structural violence (also called "indirect violence"), are, in fact, totally legal or otherwise legitimized. Johan Galtung, the scholar who popularized the conception of structural violence in 1969, felt it appropriate to also refer to the concept as social injustice, when "the violence is built into the structure and shows up as unequal power and consequently as unequal life chances." While "personal violence *shows*," according to Galtung, "structural violence is silent, it does not show—it is essentially static, it *is* the tranquil waters" (Galtung, 1969). Even the subjects of structural violence may not immediately recognize it as violence, but maybe just bad luck.

Unfortunately, the massively inequitable distribution of resources and the political and legal systems built to keep it that way are not just bad luck. They are purposeful choices. And in war zones, they are used just as cynically and deliberately as any form of direct violence could be. However, instead of individual actors (combatants) using instruments (weapons) that directly result in people killed, the violent output of structural violence is when people are killed by lack of necessities (food, shelter, medical care, education, etc.) (Köhler & Alcock, 1976). Because direct violence is easier to see, and thus measure, we often consider it the primary manifestation of war. Yet more people die from poverty, lack of food, poor living conditions, and lack of access to adequate health facilities than could ever be killed by direct violence, short of a global nuclear war.

Structural violence can be observed in political, economic, religious, cultural, and legal systems, and all forms of structural violence deprive people of their right to a full quality of life (Lee, 2019). Many of the people who suffer from structural violence don't even live in war zones but in countries with high living standards and substantial wealth. While that's another story for another book, in this chapter we'll focus on just a few of the ways structural violence is deployed and expressed in fragile and conflict-affected countries.

THE PERSISTENCE OF POVERTY

Poverty and, by extension, economic inequality are the most widely understood forms of structural violence; Galtung himself considered structurally conditioned poverty to be the first category of structural violence. Some have gone so far as to call poverty "one of the deadliest forms of violence" (Allen, 2008). How is poverty deadly? Among other reasons, poverty is one of the most significant causes of poor health in the world. Impoverished people can't afford many of the resources needed for a healthy life, like nutritious and consistent food, warm and secure shelter, and adequate sanitation services. They may engage in riskier behaviors due to lack of information or due to necessity—for example, smoking, using cookstoves indoors, or riding in vehicles without sufficient safety measures. Importantly, they can't access adequate health care for any number of reasons: they may not have the transportation; they may not be able to afford visits, screenings, or medications; or they may not be aware of health promotion and outreach efforts. They are also consistently left out of health care policy decision-making that privileges the needs of corporations (like pharmaceutical or insurance companies), interest groups, and the whims of politicians (many of whom can easily afford private care or have access to publicly funded care through their positions).

Globally, we have sufficient funds and resources for everyone to have at least a baseline acceptable standard of living, but we don't prioritize doing so. Instead, wealth has become concentrated in certain countries and among the richest individuals in those countries. Widespread economic development and other advances have ensured that global poverty has decreased significantly in the past 40 years, from nearly 42.7% in 1981 to 9.3% in 2017 (World Bank, 2021b), but it increased in 2020, largely due to the pandemic. Again, poverty is not limited to fragile countries; every wealthy and highly developed nation has some proportion of its population living in poverty. But today, more than 40% of the world's poor live in fragile or conflict-affected countries. The World Bank (2021a) expects that number to increase to 67% within the next 10 years, despite these countries holding just 10% of the world's population.

Poverty is not just a lack of income, although that is certainly a part, but also the deprivation of opportunity. Throughout this book, you'll find that poverty is a risk factor for every type of violence, from interpersonal violence in the home to all forms of collective violence. Indeed, as a comprehensive 2016 study found, "there is a causal arrow running from poverty to conflict" (Braithwaite et al., 2016). At the same time, violent conflict leads to poverty through several mechanisms, including damaging infrastructure and production (which can lead to homelessness and unemployment), destroying assets (like agricultural land, livestock, or factories), breaking up communities and social networks, forcing involuntary displacement, and disrupting financial systems, such as with inflation of the prices of goods and the devaluation of currencies (Rohwerder, 2014). Thus, poverty plays a fundamental role in what is sometimes called the "conflict trap," whereby existing conflict, through many complex mechanisms, increases the likelihood of further conflict (Hegre, Nygård, & Ræder, 2017). Further, most conflicts these days are not between nation-states but within them, and high levels of inequality between populations does seem to increase likelihood of civil wars (Baten & Mumme, 2013). When we consider the fact that there has never been more global economic inequality than there is today, this becomes great cause for concern. Inequality becomes an even greater predictor of armed conflict when the inequalities stem from disparate groupings within populations, such as ethnic or religious identities. This form of "identity group inequality" is a notable predictor of armed conflict, as can be seen in many of the most brutal wars of today (Nygård, 2018).

Eliminating poverty and economic inequality would surely not eliminate all forms of armed conflict. There is a lot of nuance in the relationship between poverty and conflict, and much more research is required (Goodhand, 2003). Further, each country has its own unique trajectory of economic development and political instability that should be considered as risk factors for poverty, inequality, and violence. At the same time, we must recognize how these risk factors interact with global systems of oppression and discrimination that affect all of us, albeit in different ways depending on our race, gender, citizenship, socioeconomic status, and any number of other personal characteristics that may increase or decrease our exposure to these broader social forces.

However, dozens of studies and reports indicate that eliminating global poverty and minimizing the vast chasm between the global rich and the global poor would not just increase quality of life for billions of people, but it would take away one of the most significant predictors of violence, including armed conflict. Many of the other forms of structural violence that we won't cover in detail here, like racism, mass incarceration, and patriarchy, are deeply rooted in principles of economic domination and discrimination that stem from or result in poverty in groups deemed less valuable than others. Humanitarian efforts that overlook genuine, just, and sustainable conflict resolution and peacebuilding initiatives (which means addressing the root causes of conflict, not just emphasizing "development" while ignoring the broken systems they live in) are not likely to meaningfully reduce either poverty or conflict, and in fact, may perpetuate both.

LEGALIZED DEPRIVATION: SANCTIONS, EMBARGOES, AND BLOCKADES AS "ALTERNATIVES TO WAR"

Poverty can affect any person in any country. For many who are currently not living in impoverished conditions, poverty, homelessness, and food insecurity are often not that far away: one lost job, one sudden medical bill, or the sudden loss of a family breadwinner can be the difference between a life above or below the poverty line. All these factors are present and exacerbated in the conflict environment. Yet there are several ways poverty is enabled and even manufactured in war zones. This is especially common against populations that are led by actors antagonistic to the more dominant actors in the international community that have the power to pull various economic levers. In this section, we will look at some of the legalized forms of structural violence that can lead to significant, often insurmountable, deprivation and poverty.

Sanctions are, simply, "the withdrawal of customary trade and financial relations for foreign- and security-policy purpose." They can include travel bans, asset freezes, arms embargoes, capital restraints, foreign aid reductions, and trade restrictions and are purportedly used to "coerce, deter, punish, or shame entities" that are seen as violating international norms or endangering the interests of those imposing the sanctions (Masters, 2019). According to the US Department of the Treasury, there are currently dozens of active sanctions programs, many focused on areas of active conflict, like Burma (Myanmar), the Central African Republic, the Democratic Republic of the Congo, Iran, Iraq, Libya, North Korea, Somalia, Sudan, South Sudan, Syria, Ukraine, and Yemen (US Department of the Treasury, 2022). Many other countries have their own sanctions programs, and the United Nations Security Council has established 30 sanctions programs since 1966, with 14 active sanctions regimes today that focus on conflict settlement, nuclear non-proliferation, and counterterrorism (UNSC, 2022).

Sanctions are often proposed as an *alternative* to war—usually meaning avoidance of direct violence. However, many critics, including public health scholars, point to the outcomes created by sanctions and argue that we should in fact consider them "a form of siege warfare" (Arya, 2008). Just as with direct violence that harms civilians, many civilians find themselves as "collateral damage" from the effects of sanctions regimes. Public health experts have, in many instances, led the charge to describe how sanctions violate the human rights of civilians in affected states, questioning the faulty assumptions that "the political gain will outweigh the human pain." In the early 1990s, for example, dozens of studies found that economic sanctions on Iraq had devastating effects on civilians, including an increase in the spread of infectious disease and an increase in infant and child mortality (Marks, 1999).

Today, many similar studies have outlined the copious ways in which economic sanctions on Iran, meant to induce regime change and quell nuclear aims, have made life extremely difficult for millions of patients, especially children and patients with conditions that require forms of nuclear medicine for diagnosis or treatment, like cancer, cardiovascular disease, and epilepsy. Economic sanctions have also increased inflation in the country, leaving many forms of treatment and therapy simply unaffordable for many Iranians (Zakavi, 2019). Importing goods like medicines is also difficult; and due to the political and economic risks, many medical entities simply won't engage with Iran. Pharmaceuticals manufactured in the United States and Europe are essentially inaccessible for most Iranians. For drugs that could be manufactured within the country, studies suggest that 50–60% are out of reach because Iran cannot import the needed starting materials. Iranian doctors are left to use older, less effective drugs with more side effects and make difficult decisions about which patients they can help and which they cannot (Massoumi & Koduri, 2015). Similar studies on the negative health impacts of sanctions have emerged from countries like Syria, Haiti, and Russia with, notably, little to no impact on the political outcomes the sanctions were meant to induce. More recently, US sanctions on countries like Afghanistan continue to lead to widespread hunger and poverty among civilians. Importantly, the elites of these countries, and those in the regimes responsible for the behaviors that sanctions are meant to punish, are often just fine, getting world-class medical care in their country that is unavailable to anyone else or maintaining the ability to travel to receive the care they need.

Taking sanctions a significant step further are instances of embargo, blockade, and siege. While an embargo is a sanction that can be enacted individually or collectively against a country, a blockade is a military operation that blocks maritime or aerial movement to or from a port or coast, while a siege is such an operation that isolates or encircles an area (Médecins Sans Frontières, 2022). There are comparatively fewer instances of blockade and siege today, and most are not long-lasting. For example, a blockade imposed on the India-Nepal border in 2015 barred most trade between the countries. As Nepal was highly dependent on import of Indian goods, including for the health sector, the effects were devastating. Suffering from shortages of fuel and essential medicines, hospitals in Nepal were forced to cease almost all service delivery except for the most dire emergencies. The price of many medicines went up, and trucks filled with much-needed medical goods were stuck at the border for months (Sharma et al., 2017).

However, this blockade lasted just a few months. Incidences of long-term embargoes, sieges, and blockades are few, but the effects are significant. Decades of research has shown how the US embargo of Cuba (not a blockade because there is no military presence preventing import/export), meant to induce regime change of the ruling Communist Party by placing extraordinary economic pressure on them, has harmed the health of Cubans by raising the price of medical supplies and food, creating nutritional deficits, and increasing rates of death from infectious disease and violence. The country responded by rationing goods and services, and their universal health system helped to mitigate some of the worst outcomes; but the negative health effects were still felt, especially by men and the elderly (Garfield & Santana, 1997). A delegation of American health experts who visited the island in 1993 felt the embargo was so detrimental to the health of the Cuban population that they called for it to be lifted entirely (Kuntz, 1994).

Perhaps one of the most infamous and long-lasting blockades of modern times is that imposed on the Gaza Strip, maintained by Israel and supported by Egypt, both of which hold the only border crossings to the territory. No airport or seaport is permitted to be built there, purportedly as a result of the 2006 election of Hamas, which is considered a terrorist organization. However, as with all such economic limitations, the people of the territory have suffered the most. There were times from 2007 to 2010 when even staples like flour, rice, and oil ran out due to import restrictions; other foods like baby formula, olive oil, chocolate, spices, and nuts were also limited at various periods of time. While the most severe restrictions on food eased over time, by then food insecurity, unemployment, and food aid dependence had increased and have never been able to recover (Gisha, 2012). Today the unemployment rate of the Gaza Strip is among the highest in the world, at 50% in 2020, due in large part to the inability to build industry because of import/export limitations. The poverty rate is also 50%, while food insecurity is a staggering 62%.

Unlike many other instances of blockade, the primary party imposing the blockade is also engaged in active warfare in the country, with multiple bombing campaigns in the past decade. In just the most recent large-scale round of bombing in May 2021, nearly 4,000 homes were partially or fully destroyed, along with dozens of factories, power plants, water treatment facilities, and health facilities. The blockade prevents import of the goods needed just for regular survival, let alone rebuilding (World Bank, 2021c). The blockade also limits medications, medical supplies, and advanced equipment needed for cancer treatment and the treatment of other chronic ailments. As a result, Palestinians, including children and the elderly, must apply for medical permits from Israel to leave Gaza and seek care in Israel, the West Bank, or nearby countries like Jordan or Egypt. Approvals can take months and may be arbitrarily denied with no explanation. Rates of approvals have plunged in recent years, reaching a low of just 54% in 2017. That same year, 54 Palestinians, including 46 with cancer, died awaiting their permit approvals (HRW, 2018). Although the West Bank is not under blockade, the ongoing military occupation there also limits the medical goods and services available, leaving many who need advanced care, like my uncle, to have to apply for these precious and often lifesaving permits.

OTHER CONSIDERATIONS OF STRUCTURAL VIOLENCE, HEALTH, AND CONFLICT

Structural violence in war does not need to come in the form of sweeping sanctions or blockades. It is often so granular, so unremarkable in its manifestation, that it goes unnoticed. Humanitarian intervention often ignores it, and political actors are rarely challenged on it. Galtung identifies many insidious ways that structural violence is used to constrain the basic needs of people, such as limiting movement, self-expression, mobilization and organizing, due process, togetherness and friendship, access to nature, and the ability to live a life of meaning and purpose (Galtung, 1975). This widespread effect contributes to the conceptualization of war as a public health crisis. Yet, because many of these outcomes are difficult to quantify, rigorous study on the many ways structural violence is used against civilian populations is lacking.

Paul Farmer, a physician and academic from Harvard University, has been widely cited as bringing the ideas of structural violence into the field of public health. In a pivotal paper, he and his coauthors note that even though many poor health outcomes are due to structural violence, it is not the role of health professionals to tackle these structural problems, and they wouldn't be able to even if they tried. But, they argue, it is vital to recognize the ways in which "social inequalities become embodied as health disparities." For example, it is not sufficient to discuss health disparities and behaviors of Native Americans or African Americans in an ahistorical context; of course, the histories of colonialism, genocide, and slavery must enter the conversation (Farmer et al., 2006). When considering health disparities, behaviors, and outcomes in contexts around the world, and especially in fragile and conflict-affected states, we must be mindful of the historic and contemporary expressions of structural violence that limit health and prevent even the most well-intentioned humanitarian interventions from making meaningful and sustainable change.

REFERENCES

Allen, J. (2008). Poverty as a form of violence: a structural perspective. *Journal of Human Behavior in the Social Environment,* 4(2–3), 45–59.

Arya, N. (2008). Economic sanctions: the kinder, gentler alternative? *Medicine, Conflict and Survival,* 24(1), 25–41.

Baten, J., & Mumme, C. (2013). Does inequality lead to civil wars? A global long-term study using anthropometric indicators (1816–1999). *European Journal of Political Economy, 32,* 56–79.

Braithwaite, A., Dasandi, N., & Hudson, D. (2016). Does poverty cause conflict? Isolating the causal origins of the conflict trap. *Conflict Management and Peace Science, 33*(1), 45–66.

Farmer, P., Nizeye, B., Stulac, S., & Keshavjee, S. (2006). Structural violence and clinical medicine. *PLoS Medicine, 3*(10), e449. https://doi.org/10.1371/journal.pmed.0030449.

Galtung, J. (1969). Violence, peace, and peace research. *Journal of Peace Research,* 6(3), 167–191.

Galtung, J. (1975). *UNESCO: interdisciplinary expert meeting on the study of the causes of violence.* https://www.transcend.org/galtung/papers/The%20Specific

%20Contribution%20of%20Peace%20Research%20to%20the%20Study %20of%20the%20Causes%20of%20Violence%20-%20Typologies.pdf.

Garfield, R., & Santana, S. (1997). The impact of the economic crisis and the US embargo on health in Cuba. *American Journal of Public Health, 87*(1), 15–20.

Gisha. (2012). *Reader: "Food consumption in the Gaza Strip—red lines."* Position paper. http://www.gisha.org/UserFiles/File/publications/redlines/redlines-position-paper-eng.pdf.

Goodhand, J. (2003). Enduring disorder and persistent poverty: a review of the linkages between war and chronic poverty. *World Development, 31*(3), 629–646. https://doi.org/10.1016/S0305-750X(03)00009-3.

Hegre, H., Nygård, H., & Ræder, R. (2017). Evaluating the scope and intensity of the conflict trap: a dynamic simulation approach. *Journal of Peace Research, 54*(2), 243–261.

Human Rights Watch (HRW). (2018). *Israel: record-low in Gaza medical permits.* https://www.hrw.org/news/2018/02/13/israel-record-low-gaza-medical -permits.

Köhler, G., & Alcock, N. (1976). An empirical table of structural violence. *Journal of Peace Research, 4*(13): 343–356.

Kuntz, D. (1994). The politics of suffering: the impact of the U.S. embargo on the health of the Cuban people. Report of a fact-finding trip to Cuba, June 6-11, 1993. *International Journal of Health Services: Planning, Administration, Evaluation, 24*(1), 161–179. https://doi.org/10.2190/L6VN-57RR-AFLK-XW90.

Lee, B. (2019). *Violence: an interdisciplinary approach to causes, consequences, and cures.* Hoboken, NJ: John Wiley & Sons.

Marks, S. (1999). Economic sanctions as human rights violations: reconciling political and public health imperatives. *American Journal of Public Health, 89*(10), 1509–1513.

Massoumi, R., & Koduri, S. (2015). Adverse effects of political sanctions on the health care system in Iran. *Journal of Global Health, 5*(2), 020302.

Masters, J. (2019). *What are economic sanctions?* Council on Foreign Relations. https://www.cfr.org/backgrounder/what-are-economic-sanctions.

Médecins Sans Frontières. (2022). *Blockade.* https://guide-humanitarian-law.org /content/article/3/blockade/.

Nygård, H. (2018). Inequality and conflict—some good news. *Development for Peace.* https://blogs.worldbank.org/dev4peace/inequality-and-conflict-some -good-news.

Rohwerder, B. (2014). *The impact of conflict on poverty.* GSDRC Helpdesk Research Report. http://gsdrc.org/docs/open/hdq1118.pdf.

Sharma, A., Mishra, S., & Kaplan, W. (2017). Trade in medicines and the public's health: a time series analysis of import disruptions during the 2015 India-Nepal border blockade. *Globalization and Health, 13*(61). https://doi.org/10.1186/s12992-017-0282-0.

United Nations Security Council (UNSC). (2022). *Sanctions.* https://www.un.org/securitycouncil/sanctions/information.

US Department of the Treasury. (2022). *Sanctions programs and country information.* https://home.treasury.gov/policy-issues/financial-sanctions/sanctions-programs-and-country-information.

World Bank. (2021a). *Poverty.* https://www.worldbank.org/en/topic/poverty/overview#1.

World Bank. (2021b). *Poverty headcount ratio at $1.90 a day (2011 PPP) (% of population).* https://data.worldbank.org/topic/poverty.

World Bank. (2021c). *The rebuilding of Gaza amid dire conditions: Damage, losses, and needs.* https://www.worldbank.org/en/news/press-release/2021/07/06/the-rebuilding-of-gaza-amid-dire-conditions-damage-losses-and-needs.

Zakavi, S. R. (2019). Economic sanctions on Iran and nuclear medicine. *Asia Oceania Journal of Nuclear Medicine and Biology, 7*(1), 1–3. https://doi.org/10.22038/AOJNMB.2018.36919.1248.

CHAPTER 6

GENDER, LIFE, AND DEATH IN WAR

Weren't men dying too young, suppressing fears and tears and their own tenderness? It seemed to me that men weren't really the enemy—they were fellow victims suffering from an outmoded masculine mystique that made them feel unnecessarily inadequate when there were no bears to kill.

—BETTY FRIEDAN, *The Feminine Mystique* (1974)

[Sexual violence] is unfortunately a very effective, cheap and silent weapon with a long-lasting effect on society. It is a way of demonstrating power and control. It inflicts fear on the whole community. It is also to send a message to the men: "You are not able to defend your women."

—MARGOT WALLSTRÖM,
UN secretary-general's special representative on sexual violence in conflict (2010)

ORIGINALLY CONCEIVED AS A CENTRALLY LOCATED base for the US Navy, Guantanamo Bay was reappropriated in 2002 as a detention camp for alleged terrorists, all men and boys, captured in the War on Terror. Since then, 800 men have been detained there, and several dozen remained there decades later, most of whom have had no criminal charges filed against them. The five prisoners of the camp that allegedly planned the 9/11 attacks have still not been brought to trial. Many of the others have been cleared for release, but politics have kept these men in this indefinite limbo on this "island outside the law" located in the south of Cuba. This military prison has since become synonymous with human rights abuses of all kinds, including physical and psychological torture (Tayler & Epstein, 2022). For the most part, the plight of these men has been largely forgotten, except for occasional comments by politicians and reports from human rights groups.

While women have not been held at Guantanamo Bay as detainees, female US service personnel have served there as prison guards. In 2005, multiple accounts from prisoners emerged that female guards and interrogators were sexually harassing the male prisoners—most of whom were Muslim and adhered to strict guidelines of gender separation—as a form of cruelty. This included rubbing against the prisoners' bodies (in one instance, an interrogator supposedly gave a detainee a lap dance against his will), watching them in the shower, and, in one incident, rubbing fake menstrual blood on a prisoner's face (*New York Times*, 2005). At the same time, other women guards at Guantanamo reported being sexually assaulted by their male colleagues or having their military careers stymied if they were seen as weak or troublesome in the face of the abuse they had to witness, enact, or endure (Mirk & Bellwood, 2014).

War is typically seen as the territory of men; indeed, most military decisions are made by men, most combatants are men (83% in the United States), and most who die of battle-related injuries are men. In general, evidence suggests that most violence is perpetrated by and against men, whether it's in war, in gangs, or in bars. However, we also recognize that the perpetration of male violence is "only one truth about men and only one truth about each man." At the same time, women, and by extension, children, are portrayed as those that suffer and are victimized, even though women can also perpetrate and support violence, and men suffer extensively as a result of violence, including those with no military involvement (Slim, 2018). The overlap of the epidemic of war with other societal ills, like sexism and patriarchy, obscures how we see men and women in war by placing them in discrete categories, usually perpetrator and victim, respectively. This prevents us from not only meeting their legitimate health needs but also understanding the complex trajectories that lead both men and women to support and participate in war or suffer as a result of it. This is a significant obstacle to our efforts to end war.

The same tired gender stereotypes that persist across all aspects of culture unfortunately also permeate our observations of war and peace. At the same time, it would be disingenuous to claim that men and women experience life and death in the war zone in the same way. As there are many types of violence in war, there are many ways to die in war. Typically, deaths in the conflict environment are classified as battle related (soldiers and civilians killed in combat) or non-battle related (increases in nonviolent mortality or criminal violence as a result of the breakdown in society). Conventional wisdom purports that while men are more likely to die from short-term, battle-related deaths, women are more likely to suffer in the long term, from lack of access to food or water, for example. While some research suggests these disparities exist, the reality is that collecting this type of data is extremely difficult. How does the epidemic of war affect men and women differently, and what does it say about war as we know it?

MEN

One of the more frightening experiences of my childhood, with summers spent in an active conflict zone, was when soldiers would come into the small village where my grandmother and most of her children (my aunts and uncles) lived, calling for all the men (they would often exclude young boys and very elderly men) to come to some meeting point in town, usually a mosque, for questioning. I would become very upset when my uncles would leave because we had all heard stories of men who did not return. What did these men do, such that every single one of them was a potential suspect of an unknown offense? My uncles, surely, had done nothing wrong! Their primary offense, I would understand later, was that they were men, and all men in such an environment, especially those of "battle age," were potential threats in the making. In many conflict-affected environments, countless men fare far worse than my uncles (who, fortunately, always came back). In the 1999 Kosovo War, for example, every Kosovo Albanian man was suspected of being a terrorist; many were immediately executed by police or paramilitary forces if captured, while others would be detained, tortured, or merely "disappeared." Accounts of similar acts of what some term "gendercide" have emerged from other war zones, including East Timor. As one study recounted, one Timorese woman was told by a member of a militia that, "you may have got your country but it will be a land full of widows" (Jones, 2000).

We've all heard the refrain "women and children first," usually in reference to life-threatening emergencies where there is a sense of urgency or insufficient resources to save everyone. Women and children, and sometimes the elderly or disabled of either gender, are seen as the more vulnerable members of society and thus as more deserving of life-saving intervention. The implicit assumption, however, is that men's lives are perhaps more disposable or that the role of men should be to stay and fight in order to allow the weaker parties to flee. In fact, the very term "civilians" has been distorted to refer primarily to women and children—those that are presumed to be innocent—ignoring the fact that women can serve as combatants and men are often noncombatants. Some men who do participate as combatants may have been recruited as children or forced into participating by being threatened with detainment or execution. But by framing men as being somehow more legitimate targets than women and children, we ignore humanitarian and political initiatives to protect men and, in effect, legitimatize attacks that primarily target men (Carpenter, 2005).

Other health risks from war, like sexual violence, are experienced primarily by women and girls but do also happen to men and boys. For example, research has found that young boys recruited as child soldiers who are raped or lose a caregiver report greater anxiety, hostility, depression, PTSD, and suicidal ideation than girls, but the issue of male rape in war is largely ignored (Betancourt et al., 2011; Johnson et al., 2008). Obscuring the fact that men can be victimized does not help women; it only limits our ability to meaningfully respond to the mental and physical needs of conflict-affected populations.

Historical evidence does suggest that, in general, men die from battle-related deaths up to 10 times more often than women do, especially men of so-called "battle age," typically between 15 and 49 years old (Ormhaug et al., 2009). Interestingly, a study of female veterans from the post-9/11 wars found that although women made up a much smaller share of the total soldiers and had a much smaller raw number of deaths, their proportion of deaths was slightly higher (Cross et al., 2011). Unfortunately, there is no comprehensive dataset and little rigorous research with which we can make gendered conclusions regarding how many more civilian men die in war than women—often, death counts of men assume that some or all of them may have been militants or had links to political factions, automatically putting them in the "combatant" category. Because men are more likely to be closer to battle or be killed, tortured, or imprisoned, the fact that more men die in the short term makes sense. But it's not just the men who suffer. Men who die in war, whether as civilians or combatants, may leave behind widows and families who depended on them for income and may therefore now face poverty and insecurity (ICRC, 2004).

Their greater proximity to battle also means that men who survive carry significant mental trauma. There are many studies that suggest that women report high rates of mental health issues during and after warfare. But typically, men face higher stigma when it comes to acknowledging and managing mental health struggles and, perhaps as a result, face significantly higher rates of suicide, alcohol abuse and alcohol-related death, and drug abuse. Rigid norms of masculinity, defined as the social rules and behaviors expected of men, lead to all kinds of other negative health effects for them and those around them. This may include perpetration of interpersonal violence, greater incidence of cardiovascular diseases, struggles with intimacy and vulnerability, greater adherence to hierarchy, and the othering of those that don't adhere to accepted norms, such as by expressing homophobia (Chatmon, 2020). Thus, it is important to recognize that the same gender norms and limitations that we regularly acknowledge harm women also harm men, including with regard to their health and well-being.

WOMEN

In any given country, women live longer than men on average, usually by about four to seven years. There are many complex environmental and biological causes for this disparity, but in most socioeconomically developed countries, men are expected to catch up to women in the coming decades (Ginter & Simko, 2013). However, in war-affected countries, the disparity narrows in the opposite direction. When considering both the short- and long-term effects of war, it is women that experience greater threats to health and well-being, especially in ethnic wars and conflicts in extremely fragile environments (Plümper & Neumayer, 2006).

Indeed, as discussed, the limited existing analysis on this topic confirms that men are more likely to die in war from proximate causes, while women are more likely to die from indirect causes in the post-conflict period (Ormhaug et al., 2009). However, much more rigorous research needs to be done on this topic, which is difficult due to the incomplete mortality data that we get from most war environments. Further, while war is primarily seen as the domain of men, health care around the world is primarily delivered by women, although they are much less likely to serve in health leadership roles than men. Health systems are often constructed in ways that ignore gender, which privileges traditional (typically male-dominated) structures of power while at the same time unofficially relying on the (often unpaid) caregiving work of women to fill in gaps left by private or public actors (Morgan et al., 2018). This means that the specific health needs of women, including reproductive and maternal health, are often overlooked.

In recent decades, many of the wars waged by the West were wrongly justified in part by the desire to "save" women from an oppressive environment, as argued by scholars like Lila Abu-Lughod. These women are portrayed as victims in need of military intervention to liberate them. Yet even in the worst circumstances, there is no event more disruptive to women and their well-being than war. Because we are much better at counting battle-related injuries and death, it is likely that we vastly undercount just how many civilians, especially women, die in the aftermath of war. We're even less adept at considering the broader impacts on the women—and by extension, their families—that survive (Bhutta et al., 2019). In nearly every culture around the world, women are expected to be the caretakers of the home and everything it entails: caring for children, the elderly, and the disabled; ensuring adequate provision of food and water; and even absorbing the anxieties and distress of their loved ones while remaining functional.

Because many conflicts occur in low- and middle-income countries where gender norms are more likely to keep a woman's work in and around the home, women are particularly vulnerable to economic shocks, like sudden unemployment in the household, homelessness, rising food prices, or devaluation of local currencies. Despite this, they are often excluded from both humanitarian and political initiatives ostensibly meant to help them (Aoláin, 2011). Women's freedom of movement is also stifled in the war environment, limiting their autonomy and ability to access health care for themselves or their children (Asi, 2021). In areas of high conflict, both men and women may support restricting a woman's access to educational opportunities or work—again, supposedly to protect them. In a study from Iraq shortly after the US invasion, half of men and women (50% and 54%, respectively) agreed that a man has the right to abuse his wife if she disobeys him (Amowitz et al., 2004). How do we even begin to unravel these dangerous gender norms, in the most fragile settings on Earth, when some proportion of women don't even agree that this is necessary?

Often, we reduce the identity of civilian women in war zones to their roles as mothers. While not all women are mothers, holding such a caregiving role in an atmosphere of violence and deprivation is particularly challenging. Aside from the immediate effects of conflict on a child, including violence, mental health issues, infectious disease, and nutritional deficits, the child's experience of conflict is also moderated through intergenerational effects, especially through the experience of their mother (Devakumar et al., 2014). Women, whether they are mothers or not, also have distinct health needs, some of which are under threat in even the most developed countries. In conflict-affected areas, however, women face unique challenges in accessing maternal and reproductive health services. The facilities themselves may be looted or destroyed; health personnel may be killed, kidnapped, or may flee; or remaining health personnel may exercise favoritism in who they will treat (Chi et al., 2015). Exposure to conflict increases the risk of maternal mortality, even for women who have more money or education (Kotsadam & Østby, 2019). In fact, 76% of countries with high maternal mortality (women who die during pregnancy or childbirth) are considered fragile states (World Health Organization, 2015).

Additionally, while war does not itself create gender-based violence, including sexual violence (which exists in all environments), it does exacerbate violence and places more women in positions of vulnerability. Indeed, rape, forced birth, forced abortion or miscarriage, genital mutilation, and other forms of sexual violence have been used as weapons of war for centuries. Who could forget the stories of the "comfort women," mostly Koreans from World War II, who were forced into sexual slavery for the Japanese army? During the Rwandan genocide, up to 250,000 women were raped; tens of thousands of women have been raped in wars in Sierra Leone, Yugoslavia, and the Democratic Republic of the Congo, and horrifying reports emerge from almost all fragile settings (Center for Reproductive Rights, 2013). There have even been reports of sexual violence perpetrated by peacekeeping troops or members of humanitarian agencies deployed to supposedly help these women.

Sexual violence committed by combatants is often part and parcel of wider aims of ethnic cleansing and dehumanization, as illustrated by the brutality of the violence these combatants display (Manjoo & McRaith, 2011). Recently, for example, hundreds of reports of rape and forced abortion came out of the Tigray region in Ethiopia; one woman, upon being gang raped by four militants who then inserted a heated metal rod into her vagina to burn her uterus, asked her captors, "What wrong have I done to you?" They responded, "You did nothing bad to us. Our problem is with your womb . . . A Tigrayan womb should never give birth" (Kassa, 2021).

These physical and mental stressors, often experienced for months or even years, take a significant toll on mental health. Dozens of studies from conflict-affected settings around the world find that women report a higher mental health burden than men, not just from conflict but also from the fragility of the postwar setting. This disparity could have several explanations: one, men are more likely to underreport their own mental health struggles; two, women are disproportionately affected by economic, political, and social disruptions; and three, in many conflict-affected countries, women are already starting from a position of disadvantage, and war and societal breakdown only magnify the struggles women already experience (Jansen, 2006). While men appear to face greater stigma in terms of acknowledging mental health issues, women face stigma as well, and their mental health is further challenged when they are unable to get their basic needs met. This does not end in the war environment; women and children make up the majority of refugees, and while they may escape direct violence and harm in their home country, they face an entirely new set of challenges in their host country, like unemployment, discrimination, and limited access to needed health care, including mental health services (Rizkalla et al., 2020).

Lastly, the role of women as combatants is frequently ignored. Women function as militants, cooks, medics, clerics, seamstresses, and in many other roles in battle, for both state actors and non-state militias. ISIS, for example, notoriously relied on a so-called "morality police" made up of women to police the behaviors of other women, search women at checkpoints, and even monitor other women captured as sex slaves. Some women may be coerced into such actions or compelled to participate to ensure their own security or access to resources like food and shelter, but not enough studies have been done to quantify the extent to which participation is voluntary. While a lot of literature exists on the effects of terrorism on women's health, very little reports on the health of women involved in terrorist activity, potentially because it is still culturally difficult to remove women from the frame of *always-victim* to *sometimes-perpetrator*.

There is, however, some reporting on the health of women in combat as service members. In the United States, there are around 200,000 women on active military duty. Interestingly, although women were implicitly barred from direct combat roles until relatively recently, women dying in combat does not reduce public support for war, as had been assumed (Cohen et al., 2020). Enlisted women describe difficulties receiving reproductive and maternal health care, experienced interpersonal violence and military sexual assault, and struggled with PTSD and other mental health struggles during and after deployment (van den Berk Clark et al., 2018). In fact, many women report leaving the military early owing to issues with family planning, long and disruptive deployments, or the culture of sexual harassment and assault. This culture can mean that women's experiences are often ignored, and they become ostracized by their male peers while they continue to have to work with, and sometimes report to, a perpetrator of sexual harassment or assault (Dickstein, 2020).

REFERENCES

Amowitz, L., Kim, G., Reis, C., Asher, J., & Iacopino, V. (2004). Human rights abuses and concerns about women's health and human rights in Southern Iraq. *JAMA, 291*(12), 1471–1479.

Aoláin, F. (2011). Women, vulnerability, and humanitarian emergencies. *Michigan Journal of Gender & Law, 18,* 1. http://scholarship.law.umn.edu/faculty _articles/71.

Asi, Y. (2021). Freedom of movement as a determinant of women's health: global analysis and commentary. *World Medical & Health Policy, 13*(4), 641–652.

Betancourt, T. S., Borisova, I. I., de la Soudière, M., & Williamson, J. (2011). Sierra Leone's child soldiers: war exposures and mental health problems by gender. *The Journal of Adolescent Health: Official Publication of the Society for Adolescent Medicine, 49*(1), 21–28. https://doi.org/10.1016/j.jadohealth.2010.09.021.

Bhutta, Z., Gaffey, M., Blanchet, K., Waldman, R., & Abbasi, K. (2019). Protecting women and children in conflict settings. *BMJ (Clinical research ed.), 364,* l1095. https://doi.org/10.1136/bmj.l1095.

Carpenter, R. (2005). "Women, children and other vulnerable groups": gender, strategic frames and the protection of civilians as a transnational issue. *International Studies Quarterly, 49*(2), 295–334.

Center for Reproductive Rights. (2013). *United Nations: women living in war-torn countries need comprehensive reproductive health services.* https://reproductive rights.org/united-nations-women-living-in-war-torn-countries-need-comp rehensive-reproductive-health-services/.

Chatmon, B. (2020). Males and mental health stigma. *American Journal of Men's Health, 14*(4). https://doi.org/10.1177/1557988320949322.

Chi, P. C., Bulage, P., Urdal, H., & Sundby, J. (2015). Perceptions of the effects of armed conflict on maternal and reproductive health services and outcomes in

Burundi and northern Uganda: a qualitative study. *BMC International Health and Human Rights 15*, 7. https://doi.org/10.1186/s12914-015-0045-z.

Cohen, D., Huff, C., & Schub, R. (2020). At war and at home: the consequences of US women combat casualties. *Journal of Conflict Resolution, 65*(4), 647–671.

Cross, J. D., Johnson, A. E., Wenke, J. C., Bosse, M. J., & Ficke, J. R. (2011). Mortality in female war veterans of operations Enduring Freedom and Iraqi Freedom. *Clinical Orthopaedics and Related Research, 469*(7), 1956–1961. https://doi.org/10.1007/s11999-011-1840-z.

Devakumar, D., Birch, M., Osrin, D., Sondorp, E., & Wells, J. (2014). The intergenerational effects of war on the health of children. *BMC Medicine, 12*, 57. https://doi.org/10.1186/1741-7015-12-57.

Dickstein, C. (2020, May 20). Women are making up more of the military, but are more likely to leave early, new report says. *Stars and Stripes.* https://www.stripes.com/theaters/us/women-are-making-up-more-of-the-military-but-are-more-likely-to-leave-early-new-report-says-1.630516.

Ginter, E., & Simko, V. (2013). Women live longer than men. *Bratislavske Lekarske Listy, 114*(2), 45–49.

International Committee of the Red Cross (ICRC). (2004). *Addressing the needs of women affected by armed conflict.* https://www.icrc.org/en/doc/assets/files/other/icrc_002_0840_women_guidance.pdf.

Jansen, G. (2006). Gender and war: the effects of armed conflict on women's health and mental health. *Affilia: Journal of Women and Social Work, 21*(2), 134–145.

Johnson, K., Asher, J., Rosborough, S., Raja, A., Panjabi, R., Beadling, C., & Lawry, L. (2008). Association of combatant status and sexual violence with health and mental health outcomes in postconflict Liberia. *JAMA, 300*(6), 676–690.

Jones, A. (2000). Gendercide and genocide. *Journal of Genocide Research, 2*(2), 185–211.

Kassa, L. (2021, April 21). "A Tigrayan womb should never give birth": rape in Tigray. *Al Jazeera.* https://www.aljazeera.com/news/2021/4/21/a-tigrayan-womb-should-never-give-birth-rape-in-ethiopia-tigray.

Kotsadam, A., & Østby, G. (2019). Armed conflict and maternal mortality: a micro-level analysis of sub-Saharan Africa, 1989–2013. *Social Science & Medicine, 239*:112526.

Manjoo, R., & McRaith, C. (2011). Gender-based violence and justice in conflict and post-conflict areas. *Cornell International Law Journal, 11*(44), 11–31.

Mirk, S., & Bellwood, L. (2014). Secret life of Gitmo's women. *Narratively.* https://narratively.com/the-secret-life-of-gitmos-women/.

Morgan, R., Ayiasi, R., Barman, D., Buzuzi, S., Ssemugabo, C., Ezumah, N., George, A., Hawkins, K., Hao, X., King, R., Liu, T., Molyneux, S., Muraya, K., Musoke, D., Nyamhanga, T., Ros, B., Tani, K., Theobald, S., Vong, S., & Waldman, L. (2018). Gendered health systems: evidence from low- and middle-income countries. *Health Research Policy and Systems, 16*(58). https://doi.org/10.1186/s12961-018-0338-5.

New York Times. (2005, July 21). The women of Guantánamo. https://www.nytimes.com/2005/07/21/opinion/the-women-of-guantnamo.html.

Ormhaug, C., Meier, P., & Hernes, H. (2009). *Armed conflict deaths disaggregated by gender.* PRIO Paper. https://www.prio.org/publications/7207.

Plümper, T., & Neumayer, E. (2006). The unequal burden of war: The effect of armed conflict on the gender gap in life expectancy. *International Organization, 60*(3), 723–754. https://doi.org/10.1017/S0020818306060231.

Rizkalla, N., Arafa, R., Mallat, N., Soudi, L., Adi, S., & Segal, S. (2020). Women in refuge: Syrian women voicing health sequelae due to war traumatic experiences and displacement challenges. *Journal of Psychosomatic Research, 129*:109909. https://doi.org/10.1016/j.jpsychores.2019.109909.

Slim, H. (2018). Masculinity and war—let's talk about it. *ICRC Humanitarian Law & Policy.* https://blogs.icrc.org/law-and-policy/2018/03/15/masculinity-and-war-let-s-talk-about-it-more/.

Tayler, L., & Epstein, E. (2022). *Legacy of the "dark side": the costs of unlawful U.S. detentions and interrogations post-9/11.* Costs of War Research Series. https://watson.brown.edu/costsofwar/files/cow/imce/papers/2022/Costs%20of%20War%20-%20Legacy%20of%20the%20%27Dark%20Side%27%20-%20Tayler%20and%20Epstein%20-%20FINAL%20Jan%209%202022.pdf.

van den Berk Clark, C., Chang, J., Servey, J., & Quinlan, J. D. (2018). Women's health and the military. *Primary Care, 45*(4), 677–686. https://doi.org/10.1016/j.pop.2018.07.006.

World Health Organization (WHO). (2015). *Trends in maternal mortality: 1990 to 2015.* https://apps.who.int/iris/bitstream/handle/10665/194254/9789241565141_eng.pdf?sequence=1.

CHAPTER 7

ATTACKS ON HEALTH CARE

Even the injured people ask us, "please don't take us to your hospital, maybe it will be targeted."

—Syrian American Medical Society medical worker from East Ghouta to the BBC (2018)

Many attacks are brushed off as mistakes, committed in the fog of war. We reject the word "mistake" . . . because throwing medical impartiality to the wind is also becoming a new norm of warfare.

—DR. JOANNE LIU,
former international president of Médecins Sans Frontières (2018)

IN SYRIA, DOZENS OF HOSPITALS and clinics have been bombed in the past decade, setting records for attacks on health care. In late November 2019, surface-to-surface rockets targeted a refugee camp in eastern Syria, killing 16, just meters from a maternity hospital whose coordinates had been specially provided to the United Nations in hopes of reducing the unprecedented number of strikes on health care facilities in the nation. Pregnant women and children were evacuated from the facility, which had been moved to the area near the camp because its previous location in Idlib had also been bombed (Kourdi & Tuysuz, 2019).

But it's not just Syria. Earlier that same year, Saudi airstrikes struck a hospital in Yemen supported by Save the Children, killing seven people, including four children. This attack, one of many in a conflict punctuated by civilian casualties, occurred four years to the day of the beginning of the war (Gladstone, 2019). During a war in the summer of 2014, the director of a hospital for the disabled and elderly in the Gaza Strip struggled to evacuate his patients prior to the hospital being bombed by the Israeli army, as many of the patients were paralyzed or in a coma (Hussein, 2014). In 2015, a US gunship fired on an MSF hospital in Kunduz, Afghanistan, for more than 30 minutes, killing 42 patients and providers (BBC, 2015).

In each of these cases and in many others, global criticism by actors such as the United Nations, the WHO, the International Committee of the Red Cross, and the MSF generally follows quickly. The safety of medical personnel and the wounded is regarded by them as sacrosanct, and transgressions as outrageous violations of the global order. While international political action has been taken to condemn these acts—notably Resolution 2286, which was passed unanimously by the UN Security Council in May 2016 after the bombing of the Al Quds Hospital in Aleppo, Syria—these attacks persist.

Perpetrators, encouraged by the lack of consequences for committing these acts, continue to target civilian health facilities and personnel. These attacks are not limited to direct bombing or raids, but also include looting or forcibly closing facilities, robbing patients, threatening or kidnapping medical personnel, and blocking or hijacking ambulances and other aid workers (Nickerson, 2015). The perpetrators' justifications may differ, but the outcomes are the same: poor population health and weakened communities. In addressing the effects of war on health, it is hard to think of a more direct effect than the targeting, whether deliberate or not, of health care facilities and workers.

THE PRECEDENTS FOR PROTECTING HEALTH IN WAR

Health is a fundamental human right. Since 1864, international humanitarian law, reinforced by the 1949 Fourth Geneva Convention, "Protection of Civilian Persons in Time of War," and the Protocols of 1977, has promised robust protection for medical personnel and facilities, as well as for the wounded. According to these provisions, an attack on a medical facility is considered a war crime if it is (a) intentional, (b) due to negligence in identifying the nature of the target, (c) a disproportionate response to a threat, or (d) undertaken without advanced warning (MSF, 2015). Protocol 1 further clarifies what may be targeted, specifying that it must be a military target that (a) contributes to an enemy's military action and (b) provides a significant military advantage with its destruction or neutralization.

In other words, only if a medical facility has been used explicitly for military action—which is, in and of itself, a violation of international humanitarian law—can this premise be violated (Sassoli, 2004). Despite all of the other protections afforded to medical facilities and civilians, perpetrators often use this justification when they target health care facilities, making it difficult for outside bodies to truly ascertain motives.

Medical neutrality was codified into international humanitarian law in the Geneva Conventions because of the long-standing recognition that targeting health care facilities and personnel for attack, theft, or partisan use is a violation of the concept of a "just war." Just war theory recognizes a war as moral only if it subscribes to one or more of the following tenets: a state defending itself, a state defending another state, or a state intervening to avert war crimes. Not only must the cause be just, but the actions as well: the action must be proportional to the injustice and must have a reasonable chance of success in its mission, and the mission must be impossible or impractical to attain through other means. Combatants on both sides are morally permitted to target each other, but civilians must be excluded from active fighting (Chehtman, 2018).

While debate continues about the overall morality of participating in war in general, as well as what national defense means in contemporary contexts, there exists an understanding that certain acts—such as torture, sexual violence, and targeting of civilians—are war crimes, regardless of their purpose or of the standing of the perpetrator (Chehtman, 2018). By these measures, harming medical facilities and workers violates all accepted notions of justifiable actions permissible in war. If this kind of attack persists, it indicates that the perpetrators believe their reasons or objectives outweigh any potential consequences. Thus, firmly worded outrage is not a sufficient response for the global community, who today can witness these attacks in extraordinary detail, thanks to modern technology and intelligence.

PERPETRATORS OF HEALTH CARE ATTACKS

Attacks on health care facilities and personnel are usually part of a wider campaign to terrorize civilian life, including bombing schools, farmland, and utilities. Despite the unique context of every wartime situation, there are several criminal and tactical causes that drive these attacks. First, they represent the degradation of social cohesion that unfurls in a setting of armed conflict, when even these protected facilities are under attack. Second, the targeting of medical facilities is often a deliberate means of waging physical and psychological warfare on opponents. Lastly, perpetrators may view medical facilities and the personnel that serve their opponents as tantamount to enemies themselves. And once a conflict has devolved to the point that medical neutrality is violated, it is often in tandem with other violations of human rights (Abu Sa'Da, Duroch, & Taithe, 2013).

One particularly troubling behavior is that of "double-tap" attacks, wherein facilities are bombed, then bombed again after first responders arrive. In some instances, a third phase targets the hospital where the wounded from the first two attacks were taken. This tactic, aside from inflicting mass casualties and psychological trauma, leads to the "bunkerization" of the remaining medical personnel, who are forced to focus on sheltering or fleeing, and so are unable to provide care (Abu Sa'Da, Duroch, & Taithe, 2013). The Syrian regime and their Russian allies have been particularly barbaric in such attacks in Syria, but double-tap bombings have also been reported in Iraq, Yemen, and the Gaza Strip.

While it is difficult to procure accurate health attack data, the WHO has been compiling data on global attacks on health care since 2014. Their data shows that, over this period, several countries sustained just a few attacks per year; but about 16 had at least 10 per year, and often dozens more. Of these countries, nine are in Africa (Central African Republic, Libya, South Sudan, Sudan, Democratic Republic of the Congo, Nigeria, Mali, Guinea, and Somalia), four are in the Middle East (Syria, the occupied Palestinian territories, Iraq, and Yemen), two are in South Asia (Pakistan and Afghanistan), and one is in Europe (Ukraine). On average since 2014, there have been about 300 attacks per year, with a large majority from Syria, and, increasingly, Ukraine. But in 2021, the most recent year of full data, there were 834 recorded attacks, resulting in 279 deaths and 424 injuries. The following year, this number was already surpassed by October, indicating a worrisome rise in the number of such attacks.

For most of these countries, the primary actors attacking health care facilities have been armed militia groups, like those affiliated with ISIS in Iraq and Libya, Boko Haram in Nigeria, Al-Shabaab in Somalia, or the Taliban in Afghanistan. These attacks are more likely to involve suicide bombers and car bombs, raids, or threats and intimidation. In some rare instances, local populations themselves may attack health facilities out of mistrust or fear. For example, misinformation about Ebola led locals to stone clinics in Guinea and attack aid workers in Sierra Leone (AP, 2014), and there have been numerous reports of violence and threats against health workers around the world during the COVID-19 pandemic.

However, state-based violence, wielding the advantage of airplanes and military weapons, can be more acutely destructive of infrastructure. Syria is a prime example, with its hundreds of devastating airstrikes by the Syrian military, often supported by Russian aircraft, which together have deployed weapons like bunker-buster bombs, which cause significant damage and high casualties. Hospitals and rescue workers are deliberately targeted in Syria's rebel-held areas by state forces, who hope to recapture the territory. Blood banks, maternity and children's hospitals, and ambulances have also been targeted in airstrikes.

While there often exists an "uncertainty of intentionality" in gauging state actors' attacks on health facilities, in countries like Syria the intentionality of targeting health care infrastructure has been made clear by the consistency of the attacks, the types of weapons used, and the locations of targeted facilities (Broidy et al., 2018). One NGO reported that health facilities are so routinely targeted in Syria that armed groups avoid meeting near them so as to avoid airstrikes on themselves (Ekzayez,

2018). Other perpetrators of state-based attacks include Israel in the West Bank and Gaza Strip, the Sudanese government in South Sudan and Sudan, Saudi Arabia in Yemen, and Russia in Ukraine.

Perpetrators, outside of terrorist groups such as ISIS and other actors with no allegiance to modern notions of justifiable combat, have become especially adept at deflecting criticism or finding ways to blame the antagonistic party. The Saudis, thought to have attacked nearly 200 medical facilities in just the first two years of the war in Yemen, often claim that their adversaries—in this case, the Houthis—exaggerate the number of their dead. They also accuse them of encouraging their fighters to attack from within civilian zones, in order to protect the combatants and maximize civilian casualties if attacked (BBC, 2017).

Other attacks by state actors have been passed off as accidents (such as the Kunduz bombing in Afghanistan) or as part of a necessary military tactic to target hidden munitions or combatants, as seen with the Israeli bombing of the Gaza Strip and Saudi bombings in Yemen. In other contexts, especially in Syria, the justification is more blatant, as when President Bashar al-Assad seeks to justify the Syrian and Russian bombing of civilian infrastructures as attempts to "clean" rebel-held areas and liberate Syria from "terrorists" (Shaheen, 2016).

IMPACT OF TARGETED ATTACKS ON HEALTH CARE FACILITIES AND PERSONNEL

Attacks on health care infrastructures have obvious consequences: the facilities are destroyed; personnel are kidnapped, killed, or flee; and civilians are left with no health care and with the knowledge that nowhere is safe. However, the deleterious impact on civilian health care from these bombings is not limited to the physical scope of the attack. Facilities in conflict-affected areas are limited to begin with, with minimal staff and supplies. Often, these health care workers are tasked with serving entire populations, of all ages and health conditions. Destroying these facilities, looting their resources, and driving out the personnel means that patients are left unserved. These populations, threatened by active violence, also become threatened by lack of basic health care services. Treatable conditions become lethal. Maternal and infant mortality increases. Children are left unvaccinated and at risk for preventable infectious disease.

In Kunduz, for example, a US bombing destroyed the only trauma center in northern Afghanistan (Cone, 2016). In Syria, where incidents of civilians being gassed, bombed, or directly attacked were reported daily, more civilians died from health care complications than as a direct result of war (Trelles et al., 2015). In Yemen, already one of the poorest and least served populations in the world, less than 45% of medical facilities are still functioning, often with limited capacity (BBC, 2017).

Aside from the loss of life and infrastructure, these types of incidents are perilous to the overall functioning of the global humanitarian aid system. In the war-torn countries where these bombings occur, social services, including health care, are often funded by donors and staffed by foreign providers affiliated with agencies such as MSF. When a donor-funded hospital is bombed, the effect is twofold: one, that specific site is destroyed, and the resources invested are lost; two, donors may be deterred from future investments in global hot spots or from partnering with actors who cannot guarantee the safety of their facilities and personnel. MSF reports that even they are unable to operate in environments that are extremely dangerous or unstable. As local health care professionals tend to flee these environments to operate in safer circumstances, this can leave a health care vacuum for remaining civilian populations (Abu Sa'Da, Duroch, & Taithe, 2013).

Additionally, global aid spending has increased exponentially, yet development in the neediest countries has not kept pace; in some instances, it has actually reversed. Contributing to this trend is that, as infrastructure is damaged, donors are tapped for short-term, immediate needs over the type of investment that would lead to long-term capacity building. They often complete these projects by bypassing local institutions, which further weakens governance and accountability in the host nation (Knack, 2013). This cycle depresses social development, creating a situation that continues to be conducive to further conflict. Lastly, health care attacks have been used in tandem with other human rights abuses to force migrations of opposition populations (Bradley, 2012).

These attacks may contribute to refugee flows that impact host countries and make post-conflict reconciliation and rebuilding more challenging.

WHERE IS THE INTERNATIONAL COMMUNITY?

In this book, we will see many examples wherein global actors who are best positioned to advocate for war-affected communities, often the most vulnerable people on Earth, remain silent for a variety of complex reasons. More accurately, they are not entirely silent, but their actions, at best, serve as public relations tools to name and shame perpetrators or actions. However, deepening the frustration of advocates around the world with the "international community's" reluctance to act on this or that issue, perhaps no failure is more perplexing than the lack of action on what should be a fairly straightforward position: punishing those who target civilian workers who are saving lives. Despite the alarming rate of continued attacks on health care infrastructure and personnel, and the condemnation by states and international bodies, there is generally little consequence for the perpetrators of these actions.

To bring attention to these issues, NGOs and other agencies have enlisted global outreach campaigns. For example, World Humanitarian Day 2017 introduced the theme of "#NotATarget," which garnered support from agencies such as MSF, the United Nations, the WHO, and the International Committee of the Red Cross. That same year, the UN secretary-general released a report about the protection of civilians in armed conflict, presenting a three-tiered approach: (a) promoting good practice in conflict by respecting international humanitarian law, (b) protecting humanitarian and medical missions as well as civilians more broadly, and (c) preventing forced displacement (United Nations, 2017). However, the UN may offer these only as recommendations, and perpetrators and their allies have continued to justify their actions or outright ignore these calls. As a result, mechanisms of accountability must be supported by all stakeholders, specifically in terms of investigations and data collection, as well as prosecutions and other penalties. This should include all occasions where health care is limited or denied due to conflict.

It is not that these protections and protocols do not exist, but that they are not enforced. Indeed, a comprehensive legal framework exists that codifies these boundaries, yet global actors too often view violations as unavoidable consequences of war (Breitegger, 2013). Currently, the only recourse available to victims and affiliated organizations is to publicize the attacks and condemn offenders, in hopes of preventing repeat occurrences. Organizations like MSF bolster their statements with photographs, videos, architectural analysis, cartography, and other techniques with which to identify perpetrators, confirm timelines, and provide an evidence base for potential investigations. However, humanitarian agencies and the thousands of victims of these attacks have no reliable avenue for justice. These attacks will persist until this paradigm changes.

The first step would be to ensure adequate investigations and data collection from incidents. Former MSF president Joanne Liu has urged the UN Security Council to conduct robust, independent, and impartial investigations of such attacks, noting that previous calls for such initiatives have been disregarded. In almost all cases where investigations are conducted, they are led and settled by the perpetrators themselves (Jones, 2016). In the Kunduz case, after the United States conducted its investigation and released a report about the incident, it called the attack an "accident." The only redress was the reprimand of 16 service personnel involved in the incident, ranging in effect from suspensions to removals, which MSF called "out of proportion to the destruction" (Gharib, 2016). Additionally, such investigations are primarily conducted when the targets are affiliated with a known agency. There is little chance that a small and unaffiliated clinic will receive the same attention.

Achieving global development goals in the sectors of health and peace requires a commitment to data collection. However, states in conflict typically have inconsistent data at best, making it difficult to hold perpetrators accountable, or to develop effective policies and prioritize resources (Gates, Nygard, & Bahgat, 2017). One reason data collection is not robust in these contexts is that it is difficult; for example, witnesses to attacks may feel unsafe about providing an accurate account or may simply not know what happened. If the information is not gathered immediately, it has the potential to be inaccurate or biased.

Some mechanisms have been developed to overcome these challenges. In Burma, researchers have developed a questionnaire for victims and witnesses to report such incidents. This could serve as a model for health workers to report their experiences and document obstacles to their medical practice for use in investigations, advocacy, and resource allocation (Haar et al., 2014).

In 1991, the Geneva Conventions established the International Humanitarian Fact Finding Commission (IHFFC) to investigate war crimes. While such mechanisms are often multilateral and are considered reliable, they are used infrequently; in fact, then-MSF president Liu called governments "too polite or afraid" to pursue them (MSF, 2015). In 2017, almost 30 years into its mandate, the IHFFC finally conducted its first independent forensic investigation, to investigate a bombing in Ukraine that killed a paramedic (Azzarello & Niederhauser, 2018).

Additionally, the IHFFC requires permission from involved parties to conduct investigations. After the Kunduz bombing, for example, the United States did not give consent to the IHFFC to investigate. Other countries have denied investigations of potential war crimes; after the 2014 war in the Gaza Strip, Israel forbade groups such as Amnesty International and the UN from entering Gaza to conduct investigations on actions that seemed to violate international humanitarian law, calling them biased (Booth, 2015). The international community must be steadfast in its efforts to investigate these incidents and override state efforts to prevent them.

Providing investigatory bodies with robust support and resources—while also shaping perceptions about what actions should be taken by states who witness atrocities in other states—would be a forceful first step in preventing these attacks and holding perpetrators accountable. Technology innovation may also play a role, as was seen in the successful use of an electronic alert system of health attacks using WhatsApp and an anonymous online reporting tool for Turkish health care organizations working in Syria. In the latter, workers would interview victims about incidents and report them to agencies such as the WHO; this allowed incidents to be verified and data to be compared and catalogued, while reducing the bias from self-reporting. At the same time, participants who feared retaliation were able to remain anonymous (Elamein et al., 2017). These reporting mechanisms demonstrate that it is not necessary to wait for fact-finding missions or other commissions to collect credible data that may be used in investigations or prosecutions.

Upon robust investigation and data collection, perpetrators may be criminally charged and prosecuted under international law. This should not be limited to individuals directly engaged in attacks, but should also extend to those who enabled such acts. In the current environment of international actors, this may seem like a tall order. Perpetrators who are, or are allied with, members of the UN Security Council could be tasked with condemning or punishing each other or even themselves.

Indeed, dealing with attacks on health care has revealed the limitations of the global order that has arisen in the post–World War II era. In one example, after NGOs reported Saudi Arabia's targeting of hospitals in Yemen and blocking aid from civilian areas, the Saudis were added to the UN list of violators of children's rights. However, they were removed from the list a week later, with the former UN secretary-general claiming that the Saudis had threatened to cut aid to the UN, a claim the Saudis denied (BBC, 2017a).

Seeing the ineffectiveness of the UN Security Council on these issues, humanitarian NGOs have sought to lead the charge. Some are calling for specialized UN action, while others, such as Oxfam, are taking a more direct approach, petitioning states to stop selling arms to countries that have used them to attack civilian infrastructure like hospitals (Gharib, 2016). Holding states accountable in other ways, such as by imposing sanctions, has also been suggested. However, advocates contend that sanctions are a form of collective punishment that primarily harm the already-fragile institutions on which civilians depend for survival: the grievous impact of sanctions on the health of civilian populations in countries like Syria and Iraq calls into question who is truly being penalized. It may be possible to punish Russia for actions in Ukraine, or Saudi Arabia for actions in Yemen, without jeopardizing civilians; but when it comes to low-resource and fragile environments where civilians already have tenuous access to needed resources, sanctions as a potential strategy most likely have utility only in very specific circumstances (Sen, Al-Faisal, & AlSaleh, 2013).

States sometimes have a just cause to enter a war with another actor. Too often, however, the war environment is used to justify actions that violate our standards of what is permissible, even in the "foggiest" of war zones. And any unwillingness of external actors to tackle the most blatant disregard of human life only shows perpetrators that there are no consequences for their actions. International humanitarian law is well understood, and exists for the purpose of preventing these types of attacks; but without the firm support of multinational organizations and individual states, these violations will continue.

We have to ensure rigorous, unbiased investigations into these incidents, and criminally charge those found to have violated laws. It shouldn't be difficult or controversial to do so. Stakeholders must be steadfast in not allowing fraudulent claims of "accidents"—or other justifications for these attacks—to outweigh their commitment to a world that is safe for civilians. If we allow hospitals to be bombed, we are also sanctioning a host of other human rights violations by suggesting that our priorities lie not with the victims but with our ties to the perpetrators and their allies.

REFERENCES

Abu Sa'Da, C., Duroch, F., & Taithe, B. (2013). Attacks on medical missions: overview of a polymorphous reality; the case of Médecins Sans Frontières. *International Review of the Red Cross, 95*(890), 309–330.

Associated Press (AP). (2014, September 24). *Ebola burial team from Red Cross attacked in Guinea.* https://www.cbc.ca/news/health/ebola-burial-team-from-red-cross-attacked-in-guinea-1.2776347.

Azzarello, C., & Niederhauser, M. (2018, January 9). The independent humanitarian fact-finding commission: has the "sleeping beauty" awoken? *ICRC Humanitarian Law & Policy.* https://blogs.icrc.org/law-and-policy/2018/01/09/the-independent-humanitarian-fact-finding-commission-has-the-sleeping-beauty-awoken/.

BBC. (2015, December 12). *US strike on Afghan Kunduz clinic "killed 42", MSF says.* http://www.bbc.com/news/world-asia-35082350.

BBC. (2017a, April 20). *Saudi "should be blacklisted" over Yemen hospital attacks.* http://www.bbc.com/news/world-middle-east-39651265.

BBC. (2017b, February 28). *Syria war: Russia and China veto sanctions.* http://www
.bbc.com/news/world-middle-east-39116854.

Booth, W. (2015, August 4). The military operation in Gaza that still haunts Israel
one year later. *The Washington Post.* https://www.washingtonpost.com/world
/the-military-operation-in-gaza-that-still-haunts-israel-one-year-later/2015
/08/03/915859a8-3480-11e5-b835-61ddaa99c73e_story.html?utm_term=.7017
f81864cf.

Bradley, M. (2012, May 7). *The crime of displacement: holding leaders accountable.*
Brookings. https://www.brookings.edu/opinions/the-crime-of-displacement
-holding-leaders-accountable/.

Breitegger, A. (2013). The legal framework applicable to insecurity and violence
affecting the delivery of health care in armed conflicts and other emergencies.
International Review of the Red Cross, 95(889), 83–127.

Broidy, C., Rubenstein, L., Roberts, L., Penney, E., Keenan, W., & Horbar, J. (2018).
Review of attacks on health care facilities in six conflicts of the past three
decades. *Conflict and Health, 12,* 19. https://doi.org/10.1186/s13031-018-0152-2.

Chehtman, A. (2018). Revisionist just war theory and the concept of war crimes.
Leiden Journal of International Law, 31, 171–194.

Cone, J. (2016, May 2). Hospitals cannot be targets in war. *Time.* http://time.com
/4314276/aleppo-hospital-attack/.

Coomarasamy, J. (2018, February 21). UN calls for ceasefire in eastern Ghouta
(Radio story). *BBC Radio 4: The World Tonight.* http://www.bbc.co.uk/prog
rammes/b09rwt5t.

Ekzayez, A. (2018, February 23). *Attacks on health care in Syria look like a bloody
strategy of forced displacement.* Chatham House. https://www.chathamhouse
.org/expert/comment/attacks-healthcare-syria-look-bloody-strategy-forced
-displacement.

Elamein, M., Bower, H., Valderama, C., Zedan, D., Rihawi, H., Almilaji, K., Abdel-
hafeez, M., Tabbal, N., Almhawish, N., Maes, S., & AbouZeid, A. (2017). Attacks
against health care in Syria, 2015–2016: results from a real-time reporting tool.
The Lancet, 390(10109), 2278–2286.

Gates, S., Nygard, H., & Bahgat, K. (2017). *Patterns of attacks on medical personnel
and facilities: SDG 3 meets SDG 16.* Peace Research Institute Oslo. https://www
.prio.org/Publications/Publication/?x=10785.

Gharib, M. (2016, September 29). Can attacks on aid workers be stopped? *NPR.*
https://www.npr.org/sections/goatsandsoda/2016/09/29/495829011/why-is
-no-one-punished-for-attacks-on-aid-workers.

Gladstone, R. (2019, March 26). Saudi airstrike said to hit Yemeni hospital as war enters year 5. *The New York Times.* https://www.nytimes.com/2019/03/26/world /middleeast/yemen-saudi-hospital-airstrike.html.

Haar, R., Footer, K., Singh, S., et al. (2014). Measurement of attacks and interferences with health care in conflict: validation of an incident reporting tool for attacks on and interferences with health care in eastern Burma. *Conflict and Health, 8*(23). http://www.conflictandhealth.com/content/8/1/23.

Hussein, S. (2014, July 16). Fear grips Israel-hit Gaza hospital. *Agence France-Presse.* https://www.yahoo.com/news/fear-grips-israel-hit-gaza-hospital-151532593 .html.

Jones, S. (2016, May 3). UN demands protection for war zone hospitals after "epidemic of attacks. *The Guardian.* https://www.theguardian.com/global-develop ment/2016/may/03/un-demands-protection-for-war-zone-hospitals-after -epidemic-of-attacks.

Knack, S. (2013). Aid and donor trust in recipient country systems. *Journal of Development Economics, 101,* 316–329.

Kourdi, E., & Tuysuz, G. (2019, November 20). Attack on Syrian camp for displaced people kills sixteen. *CNN.* https://edition.cnn.com/2019/11/20/world /qah-syria-idp-camp-intl/index.html.

Médecins Sans Frontières (MSF). (2015, October 7). *Afghanistan: enough. Even war has rules.* http://www.msf.org/en/article/afghanistan-enough-even-war-has -rules.

Médecins Sans Frontières (MSF). (2015, November 3). *Primer: protection of medical services under international humanitarian law.* https://www.msf.org/primer -protection-medical-services-under-international-humanitarian-law.

Nickerson, J. (2015). Ensuring the security of health care in conflict settings: an urgent global health concern. *CMAJ, 187*(11), E347–E348.

Sassoli, M. (2004). *Legitimate targets of attack under international humanitarian law.* Background Paper Prepared for the Informal High-Level Expert Meeting on the Reaffirmation and Development of International Humanitarian Law, Cambridge, January 27–29, 2003. http://www.humanrightsvoices.org/assets /attachments/documents/Session1.pdf.

Sen, K., Al-Faisal, W., & AlSaleh, Y. (2013). Syria: effects of conflict and sanctions on public health. *Journal of Public Health, 35*(2), 195–199.

Shaheen, K. (2016, October 14). Aleppo hospital bombed again as Assad vows to "clean" city. *The Guardian.* https://www.theguardian.com/world/2016/oct/14 /syrian-regime-bombs-hospital-again-assad-vows-clean-aleppo.

Trelles, M., Dominguez, L., Tayler-Smith, K., Kisswani, K., Zerboni, A., Vanden-borre, T., Dallatomasina, S., Rahmoun, A., & Ferir, M. (2015). Providing surgery in a war-torn context: the Médecins Sans Frontières experience in Syria. *Conflict and Health*, *9*(36). https://doi.org/10.1186/s13031-015-0064-3.

United Nations. (2017, May 10). *Report of the secretary-general on the protection of civilians in armed conflict*. http://undocs.org/S/2017/414.

World Health Organization (WHO). (2019). *Attacks on health care*. https://www.who.int/emergencies/attacks-on-health-care/en/.

CHAPTER 8

HEALTH OUTCOMES IN THE CONFLICT ENVIRONMENT

Today, the reality in too many war-torn countries is that if you don't die of shelling or fighting, you die because there is no dialysis equipment, no antibiotics, no medicine for diabetes and heart disease. Death rates by communicable and non-communicable diseases often surpass death rates by weapons. This, for us humanitarians, is an indicator that we are not confronted with mere temporary disruptions but with system disintegration.

—PETER MAURER,
president of the International Committee of the Red Cross (2016)

Necessity not only authorizes but seems to require the measure [smallpox vaccine], for should the disorder infect the Army . . . we should have more to dread from it, than from the Sword of the Enemy.

—GEORGE WASHINGTON,
commander in chief of the Continental Army (1777)

A LOOK AT THE WEAPONS of war—both the direct and the structural—makes clear just how detrimental armed conflict is to human life. But the way the story of war-related mortality is told still leaves out the bodily element. "Killed by airstrikes." "Killed by a land mine." "A widespread famine." "She suffered from PTSD." "He died in the war." In even the most detailed telling of a land mine explosion or bombed building, we are generally only informed about the number of dead and injured, with perhaps a couple of brief snippets about their identities and how they relate to the conflict that killed them. But something is happening to the body to cause death or injury. Consider the framing—"killed by airstrikes." What does this mean? This means a bomb landed in close enough proximity to a human body to render severe trauma. "War" does not kill a person—war is a political process. Some manifestation of the war, through some form of violence, provides the circumstances for injury and harm.

In arguments that war is war and health is health and never the twain shall meet, what is often lost is that mortality of any kind—whether a death from lung cancer in a hospital or a death from a drone strike—is always a health issue. We easily recognize a cigarette, a polluted spring, a sleeve of Oreos, or a car with no seat belts or airbags as risks to health and well-being. So too must we recognize bombs, deliberate starvation, and mental trauma. There is no body system that war does not negatively impact, no health ailment that war does not make worse.

Wars are becoming more concentrated in fewer countries, yes; but the way people die is also different and shows the evolution of war in more ways than one. The death toll throughout the four years of World War I was at least 20 million in multiple countries, about equally divided between combatants and civilians. Meanwhile, from the post-9/11 era to 2019, about 800,000 people were violently killed as a result of conflicts in just Iraq, Afghanistan, Syria, Yemen, and Pakistan (Crawford & Lutz, 2019). From 1990 to 2017, it is estimated that battle-related injury caused about 2.4 million deaths, as opposed to 6 million from noncommunicable disease and more than 20 million from communicable, maternal, neonatal, and nutritional diseases (Jawad, Hone, Vamos, Roderick, Sullivan, & Millett, 2020).

Aside from the effects of war on the health of civilians, however, we must also consider the health effects on combatants. It demonstrates a significant misunderstanding of human nature to assume that, in training to survive lethal circumstances or to kill other humans—and often having to carry out that training in the theater of war—the soldier or militant is not also affected mentally or physically, even if not actively harmed in combat. Yet, much of the existing literature focuses on civilian victims of war, and occasionally veterans of state armed forces. We see too few studies of actively enlisted military forces—despite the obvious physical and mental health risks of combat—let alone combatants in less formal roles. This disparity is understandable to a degree, especially with militia members: those who purposefully harm or kill those who are objectively innocent do not make for popular subjects of study. And of course, this kind of research and assessment is difficult, both in reaching populations (especially non-state militants who may be in hiding) and in getting honest answers; enlisted soldiers have strong incentives to underreport potential physical and mental struggles to maintain their career. Just as civilians are often stripped of their humanity by being portrayed as mere numbers or having their deaths discussed in terms of potential political outcomes, combatants—depending on who is doing the telling—are most often presented as either infallible heroes or irredeemable brutes. But their lives—and deaths—require understanding, too.

In understanding war (a political process) as a public health crisis, we must understand the relationship between what happens as war spreads and how it affects the human body. In this chapter, we will look at the health outcomes in the conflict environment itself; while in the next chapter, we will consider the health of those displaced by war, as well as how war negatively affects the health of those in countries not directly involved in war.

PHYSICAL HEALTH

ASSAULTS AND INJURIES

We don't know exactly how many people have suffered or died from battle-related injuries in the last century, but it's in the tens of millions, give or take a few million. Such a staggering figure is hard to comprehend, and the difficulty of collecting and verifying the data makes it even harder. Because physical injuries are the most well-recognized medical outcomes of war, we'll start with these forms of harm, even though they cause less mortality than diseases that result from war-related conditions. Looking at a graph of battle-related deaths of the post–World War II period, it's clear that they have decreased over time: spiking several times during acute periods of war, but generally receding to a lower pre-war average (Roser, 2016). Generally, we assume that combatants are the targets and civilians are harmed as "collateral damage," but evidence from many wars and other political conflicts demonstrates that civilians are in fact directly targeted.

A battle-related death is one that directly results from "the use of armed force between warring parties" (UCDP, 2021). Typically, these injuries come in the form of severe blunt force trauma to the body, causing massive blood loss, dismemberment (loss of body parts), or trauma to a vital organ (e.g., lungs, heart, or brain). These types of injuries can be caused directly by bombs and gun battles, or by their indirect damage; e.g., an airstrike causing a building to collapse and crush a survivor, or a car bomb causing a car to crash or roll over and injure the occupants. They can also be a result of torture, interpersonal violence, and other forms of direct violence, as previously discussed. Because of the countless ways of inflicting harm, the Red Cross, which operates widely in conflict-affected environments, classifies wounds not by type of weapon used but by characteristics of the wound itself: size of the wound, presence of a cavity or fracture, a vital structure injured, or the presence of metallic foreign bodies (Coupland, 2005).

With blast injuries, which are the most common cause of physical trauma in war, four levels of trauma have been identified: primary injuries due to barotrauma (injury, primarily to the ears or lungs, induced by a sudden change in air pressure); secondary injuries from debris thrown in the air due to the blast wind; tertiary injuries from people being thrown into the air or pushed into walls, cars, or other immovable objects; and quaternary injuries of all kinds, including inhalation injuries and burns (Singh et al., 2016). Outside of war zones, physicians typically are not accustomed to treating physical trauma from explosive devices and other battle-related weaponry; however, they are likely to have familiarity with gunshot wounds, which are not limited to the battlefield. For these wounds, physicians have suggested a classification system based on energy, vital structures involved, wound characteristics, fracture, and degree of contamination (Gugala & Lindsey, 2003).

Of course, often people do not die from these injuries, especially with recourse to the advanced medical care available today. However, because it is difficult to assess civilian populations immediately after injury in active combat zones, this is one of the rare areas where much of the data we have on these types of injuries (admittedly, not a lot) are from studies based on military service personnel. Interestingly, physical injuries from bombs and other terror/war-related weapons differ between types of victims: for example, while civilians have less direct exposure to battle, they are also more likely to be surprised by attacks, and will not have the protective equipment available to service personnel. Soldiers are not only more physically prepared for injury, but more psychologically equipped. Soldiers also have better infrastructure and are better prepared to deal with wounds away from medical centers, and have a greater ability to transport their injured. That said, for all victims, terrorist attacks have been found to be more lethal than war injuries, likely due to the factor of surprise and more critical injuries to the body (Peleg & Jaffe, 2010).

A study of combat wounds in American service members in Iraq and Afghanistan found that explosives accounted for about three-quarters of injuries, with only 20% from gunshot wounds (Belmont, McCriskin, Sieg, Burks, & Schoenfeld, 2012). Many survivors reported amputations, fractures, open wounds, or infections. The position of the individual in relationship to the weapon makes a great difference in the type of injury; for example, when American service members increased foot patrols in Afghanistan, we saw more leg amputations and injuries to the pelvic or abdominal regions, due to placement of roadside bombs and improvised explosive devices (IEDs) (Stewart et al., 2019).

Many of these combat injuries cause long-term damage that requires a lifetime of frequent health care—one study found that combat-injured service members reported health expenditures 30% higher than service members who had experienced injuries as civilians but not in combat (Dalton et al., 2023). In general, active combat, even without battle-related injury, leads to worse health and greater disability years later, especially if the individual is exposed to the dead and wounded (Schnittker, 2018). This indicates a psychological injury, unrelated to physical injury, which we'll look at shortly.

Even weapons that are purportedly not meant to injure or harm can have great capacity to do so—they're still weapons, after all. "Less-lethal" weapons, like rubber bullets and tear gas, have caused injuries like fractured skulls, broken jaws, ruptured testicles, damage to eyes (in some cases, resulting in eye loss or blindness) and ears, chemical irritation of eyes, skin, or lungs, and many other injuries that have led to permanent disability and sometimes death (Szabo, Hancock, McCoy, Slack, & Wagner, 2020). Often, we simply don't know how injurious these weapons can be in a conflict-affected setting; tasers, for example, have primarily been tested on healthy populations in controlled settings. Some studies, including those financed by manufacturers of the weapons, have found few adverse health outcomes in such environments. Yet in the real world, and especially in vulnerable groups, autopsy reports show that electrical weapons like tasers do contribute to death (Baliatsas et al., 2021).

FOOD AND WATER INSECURITY

Conflict is one of the primary causes of global hunger. In fact, after decades of declining global hunger, conflict has caused rates to increase in recent years. There are two mechanisms by which this happens: one, war destroys farmland, trade routes, markets, and ports; kills farmers and venders; causes high unemployment or spikes in food prices; and otherwise indirectly limits food available to civilians. Two, food may be purposefully limited or withheld as a weapon of war, causing widespread hunger (defined as undernourishment and food deprivation).

Starvation is a conscious tool of war for many depraved actors—hunger was a deliberate part of Hitler's pogroms and played an active role in the torture and murder of those imprisoned in concentration camps. Prisoners were starved, deprived of proteins and fats (which were seen as more essential to the German population), and overworked at the same time. Non-Jewish prisoners were able to occasionally receive food from outside, while Jewish inmates, the most dehumanized, were deprived (Bruaas, 2021). More recently, we've witnessed purposeful starvation in complex emergencies like those in Yemen, Ethiopia, and Syria (Dowd, 2020).

In 2021, an estimated 155 million people lived with high food insecurity, and 11 people died from hunger every minute; at least two-thirds of these people lived in countries affected by conflict. The vast majority— about 100 million—lived in Africa, followed by the Middle East and then South Asia (FSIN, 2021). What does suffering from hunger really mean? For children, it can mean wasting (a child who is too thin for their height) and stunting (a child who is too short for their age or otherwise developmentally impaired). Stunting can lead to an underdeveloped brain and increased risk of future health concerns. Both outcomes can lead to death.

While children can regain weight if given an appropriate diet, the effects of stunting are largely irreversible. Studies have found that undernourishment in childhood or adolescence can lead to many health problems later in life, like type 2 diabetes, sleep disorders, and increased risk of smoking (Mink, Boutron-Ruault, Charles, Allais, & Fagherazzi, 2020). These forms of undernourishment are highly prevalent in some of the worst humanitarian environments, including Yemen, Syria, South Sudan, Democratic Republic of the Congo, and Afghanistan (FSIN, 2021).

Adults with low body weight may suffer from severe acute malnutrition (SAM), experiencing edema (body swelling), jutting ribs, and loose skin. Those suffering from SAM are also more susceptible to infectious diseases like tuberculosis, especially children and pregnant women (WHO, 2021). Evidence observed from political prisoners and other forcibly starved individuals have found that people can remain alive, with hydration, for about four to six weeks, but eventually will die from organ failure or heart attack. In famine conditions or in concentration camps, people have been known to live for many years, but the unknown caloric intake (some days there may be greater access to food, other days none) makes it difficult to generalize these outcomes. Coupled with dehydration, an individual will die much faster—often in less than two weeks (Lieberson, 2004).

This brings us to the importance of water. Water has an interesting relationship to conflict; water shortages, especially in arid climates like Africa and the Middle East, can lead to tensions that can erupt into conflict. One database lists almost 1,000 water-based conflicts from 3000 BCE to today (Pacific Institute, 2022). Water is also an important way to track inequities. Water is the most plentiful substance on Earth, but approximately 2.2 billion people—nearly one in three—don't have access to safe or affordable water, while 4.2 billion don't have adequate access to sanitation services (WHO, 2019). The health effects of inadequate water supply (and sanitation) in conflict zones are immense: a UNICEF study found that children under five years of age are more than 20 times more likely to die from waterborne illnesses than from battle-related injury. These illnesses include diarrhea (which kills 85,000 children under the age of 15 per year), typhoid, dysentery, cholera, hepatitis A, and polio.

Water in war zones can also carry environmental toxins (mercury, arsenic, lead, cobalt, oil, soot, and even depleted uranium) and waterborne bacteria. Those who must travel long distances to retrieve water from wells or distribution sites face risk of death or sexual violence on their route (UNICEF, 2019). Desalination, a process that removes salts and other minerals to make unsafe water drinkable, is a common fixture in water-poor areas, but it also removes many valuable nutrients if the water is not otherwise supplemented. Demineralized water can also cause corrosion in pipes, which can leach copper and lead into drinking water (Zolnikov, 2013).

In indigenous communities, where access to local water has been increasingly commodified, denial of clean and accessible water can be seen as a form of structural violence. One resident recounted, "The first time the water truck brought water to my house, I thought it was a free service. When the truck operator charged me for the water, I got a real scare! I had never paid for water before." Aside from the physical ailments associated with water and food insecurity, research suggests that there is a real psychological effect of having insufficient access to these vital resources, including anxiety, depression, fear, worry, and anger (Wutich & Ragsdale, 2008).

COMMUNICABLE DISEASES

Anne Frank, perhaps the best-known victim of the Holocaust, was sent to two concentration camps in her short life. The first, Auschwitz, was a death camp, infamous for its gas chambers and other forms of torture and extermination. She stayed there for several months and survived. It was not until her transfer to the Bergen-Belsen concentration camp a few months later, in frigid temperatures and dank conditions, that Anne died. She had contracted typhus, an infectious disease caused by bacteria.

Communicable diseases have been the bane of both militaries and civilians in conflict for as long as they've existed. Smallpox outbreaks, which caused 90% of deaths during the American Revolution, prompted future President George Washington to institute the first mass military vaccination (Library of Congress, 2009). In the Civil War, the high death toll (660,000) from diseases like pneumonia, typhoid, dysentery, and malaria led these diseases to be called the "third army." In the 1990s, a cholera outbreak in Zaire killed more than 10,000 Rwandan refugees who had managed to escape the genocide in their own country.

Infectious disease flourishes anywhere there are such things as mass movement and overcrowding; poor access to clean water, sanitation, and shelter; malnutrition; or sexual violence, in the case of sexually transmitted diseases. Thus, they spread rapidly in the conflict environment. An estimated 70% of deaths in conflict-affected countries are thought to be from infectious diseases, including cholera, measles, dysentery, meningitis, typhus, tuberculosis, and HIV/AIDs. Some deadly diseases that have mostly been eliminated around the world, like malaria and polio, persist primarily in fragile and conflict-affected environments. These diseases endure not only because of poor conditions but also due to lack of vaccinations, inability to prevent disease spread, and insufficient health infrastructure to deal with infected patients (Connolly & Heymann, 2002).

The non-discriminatory nature of infectious disease, however, can spark some cooperation in conflict situations—there have been about 74 vaccination ceasefires since 1985, where warring parties recognized the risks to all from infectious disease outbreaks and temporarily ceased fighting to allow health care workers to undertake vaccination campaigns (Russell, Wise, & Badanjak, 2021). In the COVID-19 pandemic, by contrast, conflict-affected states were among the slowest to initiate vaccination campaigns, leaving large groups of unvaccinated people crowded together in poor conditions. This provides the perfect setting for the development of variants that evade our current vaccines and perpetuate infectious spread. Early in the pandemic, there were many calls for a global ceasefire, which went largely ignored.

ENVIRONMENTAL EXPOSURES

Even outside of the conflict environment—and even in wealthy and stable countries—poor, indigenous, minority, and other vulnerable groups are at highest risk for environmental threats in the form of contaminated water, air, and land. This is because they are more likely to live near industrial facilities, mines, and waste sites; to consume contaminated food and water; and to have limited access to health outreach and treatment initiatives (Gochfeld & Burger, 2011). Add war to already desperate circumstances, and the environmental threats to populations multiply, posing significant health risks to the cardiovascular, digestive, reproductive, integumentary (skin and related glands), and nervous systems.

Exposure to environmental pollutants can come from direct military action. For instance, Hellfire missiles and other types of bombs use explosives like TNT and RDX, toxic substances that can spread from soil to water. They also release metals throughout the environment, and, if used to strike water treatment, sanitation, or petrochemical sites, can spread all sorts of other hazardous particles into the air, soil, and water (Weir & Minor, 2017). During the Kosovo war in 1999, direct attacks on industrial sites led to multiple accidents that resulted in the release of many hazardous substances (Vukmirović, Unkašević, Lazić, & Tošić, 2001).

Use of nuclear weapons, aside from the initial effects of the blast, would widely scatter huge amounts of toxic pollutants, photochemical smog, and radioactive waste, causing genetic damage and increased cancer rates in the population, while contaminating food and water sources. When the US government was testing nuclear bombs and mining for needed uranium in New Mexico, local Navajo communities were exposed to uranium through bathwater and other resources. Today, the Navajo have more uranium in their bodies than any other American population, resulting in high levels of cancer and kidney failure (Brown, 2020).

Depleted uranium has also been used in armor-piercing rounds to crip-ple or destroy battle tanks, such as in the Gulf War and the Balkan War, posing a significant threat of inhalation or ingestion by both combatants and civilians (Marshall, 2007); and crew members of battle tanks are reg-ularly exposed to inhalation of substances like particulate matter, hydro-gen cyanide, and even lead.

People can also be passively affected by environmental hazards with-out any active conflict at all. To protect against insect bites, military uni-forms are typically treated with pesticides, which may cause health issues to the personnel who wear them. Military bases, of which the United States alone has nearly 800 around the world, are a well-known source of environmental pollutants due to disposed weapons, detonations, and burn pit emissions. Children who have lived near military bases in Iraq report high levels of depleted uranium products in their bodies; and those with particularly high levels, as measured by hair tests, had corre-spondingly high rates of congenital abnormalities (Savabieasfahani, Ahamadani, & Damghani, 2020).

Okinawa, Japan, where we haven't been at war in decades, is being actively polluted by its 31 US military bases, notably with chemicals from cookware and firefighting foams. These pollutants, which have seeped into spring water, local fish populations, and the fields of local farmers, are linked with multiple cancers and even with decreased vaccine re-sponse. Nearly 500,000 Okinawans rely on drinking water that has been contaminated by these pollutants, yet the US military has refused Japanese requests to inspect the bases for sources of contamination and has not helped with cleanup efforts (Mitchell, 2020).

NONCOMMUNICABLE DISEASES

Whatever the geography, political situation, or socioeconomic status of any given country in the world, the leading causes of death are nearly al-ways noncommunicable diseases, including heart attack, stroke, cancer, diabetes, and chronic lung disease. According to the WHO, they account for 70% of all deaths worldwide—about 41 million people per year. Most of these deaths (75%) occur in low- and middle-income countries. Un-like infectious diseases or direct violence, these ailments are highly influenced by individual behaviors, like smoking, lack of exercise, and poor diet (WHO, 2021). These diseases, which usually result in chronic conditions, are also incredibly expensive to treat, while making individuals more susceptible to mortality from other health risks, like influenza or COVID-19.

Conflict has a multifaceted relationship to these diseases, both for civilians and combatants, despite their ubiquity in populations across demographics. Living in the conflict environment is inherently unhealthy for many, with poor access to nutritious food and little opportunity for safe recreational exercise. Living or working in such a high-stress environment is also conducive to unhealthy behaviors like drinking and smoking, and stress itself causes inflammation that can lead to all kinds of health risks. So, while these conditions are colloquially referred to as "lifestyle" diseases, we must still recognize that many living in fragile settings do not have the option or the information to make healthier choices.

In humanitarian settings, health care access, even for the most basic traumatic injuries, is insufficient; and when it comes to noncommunicable diseases that progress over years, there are even fewer resources. On top of that, populations may be poor, have low levels of education, or even be illiterate; they may be experiencing some form of displacement or other significant life stressor; and may have little or no access to medications or monitoring devices, even if they are aware of having a health problem.

Unfortunately, as these diseases advance, the treatment options begin to narrow. In most fragile settings, what little health infrastructure exists or is accessible is unlikely to have the resources to manage or prevent noncommunicable diseases (Ngaruiya et al., 2020). In many humanitarian settings, for example, untreated diabetes is a significant contributor to amputations, while untreated heart disease leads to greater risk of myocardial infarction. Health facilities in fragile settings must often focus on treating acute needs, and don't have the capacity or resources to screen for or treat chronic ailments—from procedures as minor as taking blood pressure to significant ones like chemotherapy.

Screening may even be bypassed in humanitarian emergencies because, even if there is a diagnosis of a chronic ailment, the patient may not have access to needed care, and the clinician would not be able to help them further (Perone, 2017). Also, the unpredictability of humanitarian support from external actors, like other nations or relief agencies, means that the ability to build the health capacity that could track and treat non-communicable diseases is limited. The resource focus remains largely on infectious diseases and battle-related wounds, where intervention shows more immediate results.

MENTAL HEALTH

The Vietnam War was a turning point in our understanding of traumatic experiences and mental outcomes. Many veterans who were lucky enough to survive the war without serious injury returned home with their bodies largely intact but their minds permanently altered. Many previously affable uncles, sons, husbands, fathers, and brothers now seemed to be mere husks of themselves, inadvertently triggered by specific sounds—like a slamming door—or situations, like being in a room where they could not see the exits. They were largely unable to talk about their experiences to their families, who had not seen and could not understand the atrocities they had witnessed or, in some cases, participated in. Some even mentally blocked entire time periods, experiencing large and disturbing gaps in memory. Everyday tasks or hobbies that were previously enjoyable now seemed trivial; some men were haunted for decades until their natural deaths, while others chose to prematurely end their lives several months, years, or decades after their return home.

Not every veteran had similar experiences; many, upon returning home, largely resumed the lives they had left behind. But because the men returning from Vietnam were dispersed widely throughout the country, this picture of trauma induced by war was witnessed by many. The concept of post-traumatic stress disorder (PTSD)—a mental disorder experienced by some who have faced significant shock or trauma—had of course existed long before Vietnam. References to PTSD-like symptoms go back thousands of years, and can be found in the Book of Deuteronomy, the Epic of Gilgamesh, and the works of Hippocrates, who referred to "frightening battle dreams." More recently, it has been termed

"Soldier's Heart," "Shell Shock," "War Neurosis," or "Combat Fatigue." Notably, these terms seem to refer to the experience of combatants, not civilians. But PTSD wasn't added to the *Diagnostic and Statistical Manual of Mental Disorders* (*DSM-III*) until 1980, after nearly 700,000 Vietnam veterans required psychological support and (undoubtedly) countless others suffered in silence (Crocq, 2000).

Today, the study of mental health outcomes of war has become a robust part of the medical literature on conflict, with many studies on both civilians and veterans. Yet mental health screening and treatment facilities are insufficiently available in even the wealthiest countries in the world; they are extremely limited, if available at all, in fragile and conflict-affected countries. Though collecting and interpreting data from these settings is difficult, recent estimates suggest that about 22% of conflict-affected populations suffer from some form of mental disorder (depression, anxiety, PTSD, bipolar disorder, or schizophrenia), while about 1 in 10 (9.1%) experience moderate to severe levels of these disorders (Charlson, van Ommeren, Flaxman, Cornett, Whiteford, & Saxena, 2019).

The direct conflict certainly plays a role, but there are also the mental health effects of other aspects of conflict, like political imprisonment, and both psychological and physical torture (Willis, Chou, & Hunt, 2015). While many anecdotal reports indicate higher rates of suicide and suicide attempts in these contexts, unfortunately the empirical evidence of this relationship is lacking, potentially because of cultural or religious views about suicide and the difficulty of getting accurate data.

Regardless of the numbers, research from protracted conflicts finds that these medical diagnoses often do not capture the full scope of the mental trauma of living in these environments: e.g., what does "posttraumatic" mean, if the trauma is ongoing and the fear of death, displacement, or other life disruptions is very real, potentially over much of the life course? In these settings, mental trauma appears to be more existential, even spiritual. Residents report feeling that their spirit or future is "broken" or "destroyed," along with feelings of deep psychological exhaustion (Barber et al., 2016).

Some medical professionals and scholars have even found the concept of PTSD problematic and limiting, deeming its development as a clinical diagnosis "constructed as much from sociopolitical ideas as from psychiatric ones," particularly in the aftermath of Vietnam (Summerfield, 2001). Further, in the war environment, shouldn't it be considered quite normal and natural to have extreme mental distress as a response to brutal and desperate conditions?

In one study from war-torn Sierra Leone, a survey found that 99% of respondents would fit the criteria for a PTSD diagnosis (de Jong, Mulhern, Ford, van der Kam, & Kleber, 2000). A more recent study from the Gaza Strip found that 53% of children fit the clinical diagnosis for PTSD (El-Khodary, Samara, & Askew, 2020). Similarly high numbers have been reported across war zones and within many refugee populations. While diagnosis of PTSD clearly has some utility in certain populations, considering PTSD a mere clinical diagnosis tends to place the abnormality within the person, rather than within their circumstances. In places of active warfare with high rates of PTSD, mental health interventions aren't going to be sufficient. For genuine healing, these populations require the end of the conflicts that shatter their lives.

Experiencing or witnessing battle, torture, imprisonment, injury, or death are obvious points of trauma that may lead to increased risk of mental disorders. However, exposure to violence is just one mechanism that can lead to severe mental distress. Poor living conditions, daily hassles, domestic stress, family separation, and alcohol abuse in the family can also increase risk of mental trauma in conflict settings (de Jong et al., 2001). In fact, some research suggests that mental health interventions in conflict-affected populations are too focused on the effects of war exposure at the expense of examining the effects of daily stressors, some exacerbated by war but others that are not directly related, like poverty, unemployment, domestic violence, social marginalization, isolation, inadequate housing, and changes in family dynamics. There are also indirect pathways by which war leads to greater mental distress; for example, war exposure that provokes a parent to abuse their child may be a greater predictor of mental trauma for that child than if they had been exposed to war themselves (Miller & Rasmussen, 2010).

Lastly, although mental disorders exist everywhere, the conflict environment creates unique conditions for collective and mass trauma, including colonization, massacres, genocide, slavery, displacement, famine, bombing campaigns, and mass incarceration, among others. Aside from the individual burdens, this collective trauma can sometimes result in a collective psychological response, like mass radicalization, brainwashing, cults, suicide bombings, and other atypical behaviors that are prompted by volatile political, economic, or social environments (Musisi & Kinyanda, 2020). Many of these responses create further destabilization and community fragmentation, fostering an environment where war persists, precipitating even more trauma. It is a predictable cycle—but one that is difficult to break in environments of such low trust.

REFERENCES

Aebischer Perone, S., Martinez, E., du Mortier, S., et al. (2017). Non-communicable diseases in humanitarian settings: ten essential questions. *Conflict and Health* 11(1). https://doi.org/10.1186/s13031-017-0119-8.

Baliatsas, C., Gerbecks, J., Dückers, M. L. A., Yzermans, C. J. (2021). Human health risks of conducted electrical weapon exposure: a systematic review. *JAMA Network Open,* 4(2):e2037209. https://doi.org/10.1001/jamanetworkopen.2020 .37209.

Barber, B. K., McNeely, C. A., El Sarraj, E., Daher, M., Giacaman, R., Arafat, C., Barnes, W., & Abu Mallouh, M. (2016). Mental suffering in protracted political conflict: feeling broken or destroyed. *PLoS ONE* 11(5): e0156216. doi:10.1371/journal.pone.0156216.

Belmont, P. J., Jr., McCriskin, B. J., Sieg, R. N., Burks, R., & Schoenfeld, A. J. (2012). Combat wounds in Iraq and Afghanistan from 2005 to 2009. *Journal of Trauma and Acute Care Surgery,* 73(1), 3-12. https://doi.org/10.1097/TA.0b013e318 250bfb4.

Brown, Z. (2020). How the Navajo suffered thanks to America's nuclear weapons build up. *The National Interest.* https://nationalinterest.org/blog/buzz/how -navajo-suffered-thanks-americas-nuclear-weapons-build-166258?amp.

Bruaas, M. (2021). *Hitler's hunger plan.* Nobel Peace Center. https://www.nobel peacecenter.org/en/news/hitler-s-hungerplan.

Charlson, F., van Ommeren, M., Flaxman, A., Cornett, J., Whiteford, H., & Saxena, S. (2019). New WHO prevalence estimates of mental disorders in conflict settings: a systematic review and meta-analysis. *Lancet, 394,* 240-248.

Connolly, A., & Heymann, D. (2002). Deadly comrades: war and infectious diseases. *The Lancet, 360,* s23-s24.

Coupland, R. (2005). *The Red Cross wound classification.* https://icrcndresou rcecentre.org/wp-content/uploads/2016/04/The_Red_Cross_Wound_Class ification.pdf.

Crawford, N., & Lutz, C. (2019). *Human cost of post-9/11 wars.* Costs of War Research Series. https://watson.brown.edu/costsofwar/files/cow/imce/papers /2019/Direct%20War%20Deaths%20COW%20Estimate%20November %2013%202019%20FINAL.pdf.

Crocq, M. (2000). From shell shock and war neurosis to posttraumatic stress disorder: a history of psychotraumatology. *Dialogues in Clinical Neuroscience, 2*(1), 47–55.

Dalton, M. K., Jarman, M. P., Manful, A., Koehlmoos, T. P., Cooper, Z., Weissman, J. S., Schoenfeld, A. J. (2023). The hidden costs of war. *Annals of Surgery, 277*(1), 159–164. https://doi.org/10.1097/SLA.0000000000004844.

de Jong, J. T., Komproe, I. H., Van Ommeren, M., El Masri, M., Araya, M., Khaled, N., van De Put, W., & Somasundaram, D. (2001). Lifetime events and posttraumatic stress disorder in 4 postconflict settings. *JAMA, 286*(5), 555–562. https:// doi.org/10.1001/jama.286.5.555.

de Jong, K., Mulhern, M., Ford, N., van der Kam, S., & Kleber, R. (2000). The trauma of war in Sierra Leone. *Lancet, 355*(9220), 2067–2068. https://doi.org/10 .1016/S0140-6736(00)02364-3.

Dowd, C. (2020). Conflict and hunger. In *The Palgrave Encyclopedia of Peace and Conflict Studies.* https://doi.org/10.1007/978-3-030-11795-5_161-1.

El-Khodary, B., Samara, M., & Askew, C. (2020). Traumatic events and PTSD among Palestinian children and adolescents: the effect of demographic and socioeconomic factors. *Frontiers in Psychiatry, 11.* https://doi.org/10.3389/fpsyt .2020.00004.

Food Security Information Network (FSIN). (2021). *Global report on food crises.* https://docs.wfp.org/api/documents/WFP-0000127343/download/?_ga=2 .174232162.1315345602.1624185147-659202006.1615888715.

Gochfeld, M., & Burger, J. (2011). Disproportionate exposures in environmental justice and other populations: the importance of outliers. *American Journal of Public Health, 101* (Suppl 1), S53–S63. https://doi.org/10.2105/AJPH.2011.300121.

Gugala, Z., & Lindsey, R. (2003). Classification of gunshot injuries in civilians. *Clinical Orthopaedics and Related Research, 408,* 65–81.

Jawad, M., Hone, T., Vamos, E., Roderick, P., Sullivan, R., & Millett, C. (2020). Estimating indirect mortality impacts of armed conflict in civilian populations: panel regression analyses of 193 countries, 1990–2017. *BMC Medicine, 18.*

Library of Congress (LoC). (2009). *George Washington and the first mass military inoculation.* https://www.loc.gov/rr/scitech/GW&smallpoxinoculation.html.

Lieberson, A. (2004). How long can a person survive without food? *Scientific American.* https://www.scientificamerican.com/article/how-long-can-a-person-survive-without-food/.

Marshall, A. (2007). Gulf War depleted uranium risks. *Journal of Exposure Science & Environmental Epidemiology, 18,* 95–108.

Miller, K., & Rasmussen, A. (2010). War exposure, daily stressors, and mental health in conflict and post-conflict settings: bridging the divide between trauma-focused and psychosocial frameworks. *Social Science & Medicine, 70,* 7–16.

Mink, J., Boutron-Ruault, M. C., Charles, M. A., et al. (2020). Associations between early-life food deprivation during World War II and risk of hypertension and type 2 diabetes at adulthood. *Scientific Reports, 10,* 5741. https://doi.org/10.1038/s41598-020-62576-w.

Mitchell, J. (2020). US military bases are poisoning Okinawa. *The Diplomat.* https://thediplomat.com/2020/10/us-military-bases-are-poisoning-okinawa/.

Musisi, S., & Kinyanda, E. (2020). Long-term impact of war, civil war, and persecution in civilian populations—conflict and post-traumatic stress in African communities. *Frontiers in Psychiatry, 11*(20). https://doi.org/10.3389/fpsyt.2020.00020.

Ngaruiya, C., Bernstein, R., Leff, R., Wallace, L., Agrawal, P., Selvam, A., Hersey, D., & Hayward, A. (2020). Systematic review on chronic non-communicable disease in disaster settings. *medRxiv.* https://doi.org/10.1101/2020.10.15.20213025.

Norman, R. E., Byambaa, M., De, R., Butchart, A., Scott, J., et al. (2012). The long-term health consequences of child physical abuse, emotional abuse, and neglect: a systematic review and meta-analysis. *PLOS Medicine 9*(11), e1001349. https://doi.org/10.1371/journal.pmed.1001349.

Pacific Institute. (2022). *Water conflict chronology.* http://www.worldwater.org/conflict/list/.

Peleg, K., Jaffe, D. H., & Israel Trauma Group (2010). Are injuries from terror and war similar? A comparison study of civilians and soldiers. *Annals of Surgery, 252*(2), 363–369. https://doi.org/10.1097/SLA.0b013e3181e98588.

Roser, M. (2016). War and peace. *Our World in Data.* https://ourworldindata.org/war-and-Peace.

Russell, I., Wise, L., & Badanjak, S. (2021). VaxxPax: a dataset of vaccination ceasefires, 1985–2018 [dataset]. University of Edinburgh Law School. https://doi.org/10.7488/ds/3131.

Savabieasfahani, M., Ahamadani, F., & Damghani, A. (2020). Living near an active U.S. military base in Iraq is associated with significantly higher hair thorium and increased likelihood of congenital anomalies in infants and children. *Environmental Pollution, 256,* 113070. https://doi.org/10.1016/j.envpol.2019.113070.

Schnittker, J. (2018). Scars: the long-term effects of combat exposure on health. *Socius: Sociological Research for a Dynamic World, 4.* https://doi.org/10.1177/2378023118813017.

Singh, A. K., Ditkofsky, N. G., York, J. D., Abujudeh, H. H., Avery, L. A., Brunner, J. F., Sodickson, A. D., & Lev, M. H. (2016). Blast injuries: from improvised explosive device blasts to the Boston Marathon bombing. *Radiographics: A Review Publication of the Radiological Society of North America, 36*(1), 295–307. https://doi.org/10.1148/rg.2016150114.

Stewart, L., Shaikh, F., Bradley, W., Lu, D., Blyth, D., Petfield, J., Whitman, T., Krauss, M., Greenberg, L., & Tribble, D. (2019). Combat-related extremity wounds: injury factors predicting early onset infections. *Military Medicine, 184*(1), 83–91. https://doi.org/10.1093/milmed/usy336.

Summerfield, D. (2001). The invention of post-traumatic stress disorder and the social usefulness of a psychiatric category. *BMJ, 322*(7278): 95–98.

Szabo, L., Hancock, J., McCoy, K., Slack, D., & Wagner, D. (2020). Fractured skulls, lost eyes: police break their own rules when shooting protesters with "rubber bullets." *USA Today.* https://www.usatoday.com/in-depth/news/nation/2020/06/19/police-break-rules-shooting-protesters-rubber-bullets-less-lethal-projectiles/3211421001/.

UNICEF. (2019). More children killed by unsafe water, than bullets, says UNICEF chief. *UN News.* https://news.un.org/en/story/2019/03/1035171.

Uppsala Conflict Data Program (UCDP). (2021). *UCDP definitions.* https://www.pcr.uu.se/research/ucdp/definitions.

Vukmirović, Z., Unkašević, M., Lazić, L., & Tošić, I. (2001). Regional air pollution caused by a simultaneous destruction of major industrial sources in a war zone. The case of April Serbia in 1999. *Atmospheric Environment, 35*(15), 2773–2782.

Weir, D., & Minor, E. (2017). *The environmental consequences of the use of armed drones.* Conflict and Environment Observatory. https://ceobs.org/the-environmental-consequences-of-the-use-of-armed-drones/.

Willis, S., Chou, S., & Hunt, N. (2015). A systematic review on the effect of political imprisonment on mental health. *Aggression and Violent Behavior, 25,* 173–183.

World Health Organization (WHO). (2019a). Management of severe acute malnutrition in individuals with active tuberculosis. *e-Library of Evidence for Nutrition Actions (eLENA)*. https://www.who.int/elena/titles/sam_tuberculosis/en/.

World Health Organization (WHO). (2019b). *1 in 3 people globally do not have access to safe drinking water—UNICEF, WHO*. https://www.who.int/news/item/18-06-2019-1-in-3-people-globally-do-not-have-access-to-safe-drinking-water-unicef-who.

World Health Organization (WHO). (2021). *Noncommunicable diseases*. https://www.who.int/health-topics/noncommunicable-diseases#tab=tab_1.

Wutich, A., & Ragsdale, K. (2008). Water insecurity and emotional distress: coping with supply, access, and seasonal variability of water in a Bolivian squatter settlement. *Social Science & Medicine, 67*, 2116–2125.

Zolnikov, T. R. (2013). The maladies of water and war: addressing poor water quality in Iraq. *American Journal of Public Health, 103*(6), 980–987. https://doi.org/10.2105/AJPH.2012.301118.

CHAPTER 9

THE HEALTH EFFECTS OF WAR AT HOME

Significantly, war does not simply involve the arena of combat. Wars are supported by individuals on a number of fronts. Ideologically, most of us have been raised to believe war is necessary and inevitable. In our daily lives, individuals who have passively accepted this socialization reinforce value systems that support, encourage, and accept violence as a means of social control. Such acceptance is a prerequisite for participation in imperialist struggle and for supporting the militarism that aids such struggle.

—BELL HOOKS, *Feminism and Militarism: A Comment* (1995)

You know, it's funny when it rains it pours
They got money for wars, but can't feed the poor
Said it ain't no hope for the youth and the truth is
It ain't no hope for the future.

—TUPAC SHAKUR, "Keep Ya Head Up" (1993)

WE'VE LEARNED QUITE A few things about infectious disease, epidemics, and pandemics in the past few years. Maybe too much. First, obviously, if disease is given the opportunity to spread, it does, especially if the mechanisms to prevent its spread are politicized and misinformation becomes rampant. Second, while the disease may be the same everywhere, the outcomes differ depending on a variety of factors: socioeconomic status, gender, age, citizenship, employment, preexisting health conditions, and many more.

To understand war as a public health crisis, we must recognize that the effects of war are not limited to the battlefield or even to those communities that are directly involved. This misconception leads those of us who live in relatively stable and wealthy nations to assume that while war is certainly bad, it's surely not a public health emergency for the rest of us—how could it be? Most people reading this are unlikely to be living in a fragile or conflict-affected area. Most people have never served in the armed forces. The health effects of war are terrible, surely, but they're limited to the war environment. How is war a public health threat, let alone the most significant health threat, to a citizen of a country where war isn't being waged?

In the midst of the worst public health crisis in living memory, I found it ironic and slightly disheartening to read that some of the world's wealthiest countries, including several with universal health care, were relying on military personnel and the arms industry to deal with the strain on the health system. The British requested field hospitals to be built by Marshall Aerospace and Defence on behalf of the Ministry of Defence, while the United States deployed thousands of military medical personnel to support overwhelmed hospitals, and invoked the Defense Production Act to manufacture at-home test kits in light of a national shortage. In Israel, some defense contractors shifted to producing technologies useful for doctors and hospitals. "We're very good at the war sciences and war technology, and this is a war," said a hospital administrator in Haifa. "We need to take the technologies we use in war and implement them on the medical battlefield" (Shpigel, 2020).

The disparity in what we need, as opposed to what we're given, is never clearer than when there is an emergency. At such times, the typical assumptions that undergird so much of our societies' functioning are laid bare. The debacle of the US pull-out from Afghanistan in 2021, buoyed by billions in military spending and thousands of lost lives, juxtaposed with the utter global failure to manage the COVID-19 pandemic, led many to rethink exactly what we're getting in the name of so-called "national security." In this chapter, I'll address not only the health outcomes of war far away from battle—both for those who return from war as veterans and for those who escape war—but also the costs of building a society around an unquestioned principle of militarism. Why do we live this way? Do we have to?

THE HEALTH OUTCOMES OF WAR, AT HOME: VETERANS

Famously, the United States does not have universal health care. For veterans of the American armed forces, however, there is something that at least resembles a universal system. While not every veteran is eligible for health services through Veterans Affairs (VA), most who have served for at least two years, without a dishonorable discharge, can apply for VA health benefits. Those who were discharged with a disability, recently served in combat, were a prisoner of war, or received any number of honors (such as a Purple Heart or Medal of Honor) receive higher priority for these benefits.

The VA operates the largest health system in the country, and about nine million veterans receive VA benefits. In 2002, the VA spent about $35 billion on medical care. In 2019, with the increasing average age of veterans and their more complex health needs, including severe disabilities from combat injuries, the price tag for medical care reached nearly $80 billion (USAFacts, 2021). Just for veterans of the post-9/11 wars, estimated health care costs will reach up to $2.5 trillion by 2050. However, these significant costs are often not included in war budgeting, and there are no financial provisions to set aside the needed funds, as there are for programs such as Social Security or Medicare (Bilmes, 2021).

VA benefits are an often-lauded part of the US federal budget. What could be more honorable than serving the health needs of those men and women who risked their lives, far away from the comforts of home, for American interests? It's important to remember, however, that the reason American veterans need a specialized health care system is because there is, again, no universal health care system in the United States. Thus, many veterans fall through the cracks. A recent study found that about 1.5 million veterans are uninsured, and two million skip needed care because they can't afford it. These veterans, including many with chronic ailments like heart disease, are less likely to receive needed immunizations or even an annual physical exam (Gaffney, Himmelstein, & Woolhandler, 2020).

Despite the VA's ever-inflating budget, it receives proportionally less funding than is provided to private medical providers. VA doctors earn less than doctors in the private sector and, because of the nature of the Federal Government budgetary process, they may experience unexpected salary freezes or budget cuts, which can push them out of federal service. VA hospitals are not equitably distributed to all parts of the country where most veterans live, so many veterans with VA benefits may not have access to a nearby VA facility. Lastly, some wish to privatize the VA by essentially using it to purchase private insurance for veterans to seek health care on their own. Veterans' groups and politicians from both major political parties argue that this would have negative health impacts on veterans (Lachmann, 2018).

Aside from the typical health needs associated with growing older, many veterans have suffered significant combat injuries, such as burns, broken bones, traumatic brain injuries, paralysis, loss of sight or hearing, loss of limbs, and combat-related mental health disorders, including post-traumatic stress disorder (PTSD). Many other health issues go understudied, like the effects of long-term exposure to burn pits, heatstroke, and suicide attempts, both in theater and back at home. Due to the difficulties of transitioning back to civilian life, veterans also face higher risks of substance and alcohol abuse. The health outcomes of private contractors who work with the military, especially those who are not US citizens, are consistently underreported, leaving an entire population out of our calculation of just how harmful war can be (Costs of War, 2021). While most studies related to the health outcomes of veterans focus on the US Armed Forces, similar trends have been seen in militaries around the world.

Of course, most service members don't do it alone. They are often supported by families who are expected to make significant sacrifices, including living through multiple deployments. In fact, many military families and members of the armed forces report that long deployments are the most stressful aspect of life in the military. These periods of family separation, which can last for months or even up to a year, are incredibly stressful, resulting in more depressive symptoms in service members, higher rates of suicide, and greater anxiety (and even PTSD) in spouses.

Children report more mental health distress as well, and greater incidence of behavioral problems. And those are just the results of the separation itself—when the military member is injured or experiences physical or mental trauma as a result of combat, the risk for PTSD and depression is even greater. Post deployment, the service member may experience greater psychological and physical aggression. Family cohesion becomes more fragile, and risk of divorce increases, while relationship quality between children and their parents, even the non-deployed parent, can deteriorate as well (Meadows et al., 2016).

THE HEALTH OF THOSE FINDING A NEW HOME: REFUGEES

We've addressed a lot of staggering statistics throughout the course of this book, but here's one that I think we really need to keep an eye on in coming years, as it's likely to increase significantly as threats to people's homes (from ongoing conflict and, increasingly, climate change) increase. As of mid-2022, at least 89.3 million people worldwide have been forcibly displaced. Of these people, about 27 million are refugees, and 4.6 million are seeking asylum (meaning they have fled persecution in their home country but have not yet been given official status). Nearly 70% of these people are from just five countries—Syria, Venezuela, Afghanistan, South Sudan, and Myanmar—and about 40% are hosted in another five countries: Turkey, Colombia, Uganda, Pakistan, and Germany. Nearly half (42%) of existing refugees are children, and nearly one million children were born as refugees (UNHCR, 2022).

Because many refugees are undocumented and use unofficial (and often very dangerous) channels to cross borders, we know that these figures underestimate just how many there are. Further, people who leave their homes due to increasing temperatures or rising sea levels, generally termed "climate refugees," don't meet our current criteria for refugee status and aren't included in these counts.

As the UN High Commissioner for Refugees puts it, "No one becomes a refugee by choice." Many refugees attempt to stay in even the worst war-torn conditions for as long as possible, especially the poor, elderly, and those for whom movement is difficult for some other reason. Just consider the thought process behind leaving your home, your belongings, maybe even some loved ones, without knowing if you will ever return. Couple that difficult decision with the knowledge that in many host countries, refugees are dehumanized and even demonized. They are sometimes disparaged in the media or by politicians as barbarians—potentially even enemies!—trying to take advantage of the system, even though seeking asylum is a human right. This plays into the prejudices of many citizens of host nations, who in turn demand less generous treatment of refugees (Esses, Veenvliet, Hodson, & Mihic, 2008).

At the same time, host countries that cannot fully meet the health needs of their refugee populations face an increased burden on their own health systems, which can lead to unintended economic, political, and social consequences for local communities and governments (Dator, Abunab, & Dao-ayen, 2018). Refugees may not know how to access care or interpret results, and may have difficulties with making appointments, understanding diagnostic or screening tests, or reconciling the treatment they receive with their expectations (for example, not being able to get antibiotics that were commonly available in their home country) (Cheng, Drillich, & Schattner, 2015). Some refugees even face discrimination or hostility from health care workers in host countries due to language barriers, accents, or their race. Thus, it's not just health care they need, but culturally appropriate health care delivered by competent professionals (Mangrio & Forss, 2017).

Refugees, especially those living in camps, are often exposed to incredibly poor living conditions—e.g., crowding, and limited access to water, sanitation, and hygiene—and often face language and legal barriers to accessing services in their host country. They face a higher risk of both communicable and noncommunicable disease—especially if their home country had poor health infrastructure—as well as related risk factors like smoking and poor diet, and may not even know their health status upon leaving their home country. Yet, such is the burden placed on host country health systems (many of which are middle-income countries themselves) that, if refugees are able to receive health care at all, it will likely focus more on their acute needs than on those that require long-term treatment and monitoring (Al-Oraibi, Nellums, & Chattopadhyay, 2021).

Refugees' high dependence on humanitarian aid, and especially food aid, for months or even years at a time, leaves them at risk for macro- and micronutrient deficiencies, like anemia, iron deficiency, iodine deficiency, beriberi (vitamin B-1 deficiency), and even scurvy (vitamin C deficiency) (Dye, 2007). Those exposed to violence, discrimination, or other threats in their home countries are more likely to experience mental health challenges, but the process of becoming a refugee is stressful no matter the circumstances. Unfortunately, refugees face significant stigma associated with seeking treatment for mental health issues, if these services are available to them at all. Their home country may have been repressive, or have upheld a culture where mental health was ignored; they may be afraid to share their struggles, or feel shameful about them; or they may not see the benefits in talking about their experiences and challenges (Shannon, Wieling, Simmelink-McCleary, & Becher, 2014).

While it is clear that refugees bring a panoply of health needs with them, we also tend to obscure their diversity—they're just "refugees." But of course, the health status they arrive with is highly dependent on all the social determinants of health they experienced before they left. Are they young or old, rich or poor? Did they leave a country with some semblance of a health system, or are they escaping a country with a decimated health system? There are certainly areas of intersectionality in terms of health needs, but unless we recognize that refugees, like any other disparate grouping of people, require targeted interventions, we will miss important ways to help them integrate into their new communities and remain healthy (Barnes, Harrison, & Heneghan, 2004).

Monitoring the health of refugees isn't just vital to their own well-being—it serves the health of their host countries as well. In 2021, refugee flights from Afghanistan were temporarily paused after a few were diagnosed with measles, and others who had entered the United States and been housed in military bases in Virginia and Wisconsin were diagnosed with measles upon arrival (Finley, 2021). For those refugees fortunate enough to return home (which many increasingly do not), they are likely to go back to a country with a broken health care system, a destroyed infrastructure, and significant health worker shortages (UN, 2019).

THE HEALTH OF THOSE NOT SO FAR FROM HOME: INTERNALLY DISPLACED PEOPLE

"In the spring of 2012, the way to leave Sabinah opened because the Syrian army was coming and they wanted to evacuate the town. We hurried out in our little car with only our dirty clothes, our documents, and our memories. Because my family was so large, we had to split into four groups, each going to a different relative throughout Syria, as nobody could afford to take us all in." So begins the story of a 23-year-old Syrian man who wrote about his journey away from home—a story that resembles those of millions of other refugees (Awwadawnan, 2018). Weeks or months of waiting, all the while witnessing the deterioration of their community. Stressful discussions and unfathomable choices. A decision, a few packed precious belongings, and a prayer to return, someday. Then, escape. Ultimately, this man ended up in a refugee camp in Greece. But his story began as an internally displaced person (IDP), i.e., someone who has fled their home due to violence, human rights violations, or disaster, but has not crossed an international border. IDPs, like refugees, escape home when it is no longer safe; but unlike refugees, they are unable or unwilling to leave their home country altogether.

In 2022, the number of IDPs reached a high of nearly 60 million people—almost double the number of refugees. In 2021 alone, 14 million more people were internally displaced due to conflict; most were in Ethiopia, the Democratic Republic of the Congo, Afghanistan, and Myanmar, and millions more were internally displaced in Ukraine in 2022. Yet most internal displacement has been due to disasters, primarily from weather-related events. Even countries not affected by conflict, like China and India, reported millions of IDPs in 2021 (IDMC, 2022). Unlike the global refugee population, which is about evenly split between males and females, it is estimated that about 80% of IDPs are women and children (Amodu, Richter, and Salami, 2020).

Also, unlike refugees, who have internationally recognized rights and protections, IDPs do not have a special legal status and remain under the authority of their home country's government, even if that government is the one threatening their home to begin with. External actors are more hesitant to become involved with IDP populations, due to norms and guidelines regarding intervention within another sovereign state. Further, though the United Nations developed the Guiding Principles on Internal Displacement in 1998, they are not binding. Instead, they are a series of provisions rooted in existing international law that often rely too heavily on the assumption that a citizen of a country (which an IDP remains, in theory) should be able to depend on their government to guarantee their human rights—including access to food, water, and health care (Cohen, 1999). While many multilateral agencies and countries have embraced these guidelines, and some states with IDP populations have utilized them, some of the worst global actors have pushed back against the provisions or disregarded them altogether.

In some ways, IDPs have the worst of all worlds: they have fled their homes, facing the same precarity as many refugees, but they remain closer to the violence and conflict they fled initially. They don't have the same level of international attention and support, they are harder to access and identify, and they remain dependent on whatever services their country makes available to them. If they have family or friends in the country, that might offer them some comfort and reprieve; but in countries where poverty is widespread, or where fighting moves throughout different regions, the ability of IDPs to find a safe and permanent residence is limited. In fact, the data tells us that some IDPs report worse mental health outcomes than those who are externally displaced—particularly those IDPs left in politically or economically unstable countries (Haslam, 2005).

IDPs are also more likely to experience extreme poverty, and although they remain citizens of their home country, they suffer death and disease at rates higher than their country baseline. Large population shifts within nations also burden health facilities in the regions to which people migrate, straining available resources in the host communities (Cantor et al., 2021).

THE HEALTH OF THE REST OF US: LIVING IN A MILITARIZED CULTURE

Okay, so you're lucky enough not to live in, or be escaping, a war zone—and you're not in the military or related to someone in active service. Surely, you're in the clear, right? Unfortunately, no.

You may not be at high risk of airstrikes, but propaganda is another matter: you could be forgiven if you've vastly overestimated your likelihood of being killed by a terrorist attack, especially in the post-9/11 era. After the attacks on the World Trade Center, politicians and supposed analysts blanketed cable news and op-ed sections with warnings about the risks of terrorism, especially from Islamic militants. Rather than using evidence and credible data, they relied on emotional language and unsubstantiated conjecture, along with overt racism. But when it comes from the mouth of a well-known figure, it can sound pretty convincing to an audience that is otherwise relatively uninformed on such issues. Terrorist attacks perpetrated by the perceived enemy of the moment, Muslims, received 375% more attention than those perpetrated by non-Muslims. But only 2.6% of terrorist attacks take place in Western countries—the vast majority of victims of Islamic terrorists and armed groups, including the Taliban and ISIS, were other Muslims, in their own countries; yet these victims were often painted as complicit in their own misery.

In reality, terrorism was much more common in the West in the 1970s and 1980s, and was mostly perpetrated by domestic actors. Although the threat of terrorism remains exponentially small, the number of news articles or segments about terrorism has increased significantly over the past two decades (Ahmad, 2021). This is how the seed of militarism gets planted: you (the citizen) are always under threat, and to combat that threat, we (the state or a non-state militia) need to engage in violence, dehumanization, and isolation, while deprioritizing other human needs like shelter, health care, and food. The threat of imminent violence, and the justification of state violence to "protect," becomes normalized, and accountability mechanisms begin to be seen as obstacles and restrictions to overcome, rather than as vital safeguards of our national values and principles.

This normalization can happen quickly, especially if supported by political elites. Just look at the aftermath of 9/11 in the United States: much of the public accepted a significant overhaul of domestic surveillance and full-throttle investment into foreign military action, purportedly to ensure safety and security. Those who argued against it, or merely questioned it, were largely resisted or ignored. In the United States, this meant accepting warrantless surveillance and raids on homes, as well as the expansion of the Foreign Intelligence Surveillance Act Court, which operates in secret and enables targeting of suspects with much less evidence than traditional courts. The president's war powers were also significantly enhanced, meaning that the same Authorization for the Use of Military Force that was passed shortly after 9/11 is still used to justify military action throughout the Middle East and Africa, with no public accountability or congressional debate. Despite ongoing evidence of countless "mistakes" or high rates of "collateral damage" (i.e., innocent people being killed), support for drone strikes remains high in the United States, potentially because the media consistently underreports the numbers and identities of the dead.

Militarism is also present in shaping the narrative of a conflict, for example, as to which eyewitness accounts are privileged and disseminated. Most often, official sources—spokespeople for the governments and militaries that carried out the attacks—are preferred over the accounts of witnesses on the ground (Ahmad, 2015). In the UK, attacks on civilians in countries like Syria have been so normalized that less than half of all British citizens believe that such attacks are newsworthy. This underscores a disturbing trend—the more war crimes and atrocities that are committed, the more normal they seem, and the more disconnected from them external populations feel; even if their own governments are implicitly or explicitly enabling these violations (Syria Relief, 2021). This acceptance and normalization of violence, discrimination, and disregard for human life, whether through passive or active means, seem to be obvious evidence of these societies' deeply skewed priorities.

Militarism has been defined in many ways in different disciplines throughout history, although the term became more prominent in the twentieth century, as militaries became more permanent fixtures of society. One comprehensive definition, useful to the framing of militarism as directly opposed to well-being, is "the extension of military influence into civilian social, political, and economic spheres, with the associated prioritizing, promotion, and preservation of a nation's armed forces" (Woodward, 2009).

Prominent feminist scholar Cynthia Enloe takes the concept further, arguing that *militarism* is the *belief* that some (usually men) are natural protectors, and that others (often women) should be grateful for their protection; that soldiers, above other contributors to society, deserve special praise; that it is natural to have enemies; and that physical force, over other forms of human interaction, is the optimal way to resolve disputes. Meanwhile, *militarization* is the *process* by which the beliefs of militarism are absorbed by a society—through the history that is taught, the way children are raised, the media that is presented, the expectations of gender norms, and the division of a government's budget (Enloe, 2016).

Contemporary conversations about these phenomena typically include critique of the creeping militarization in policing. In some countries, like Nepal and the Philippines, the military plays an official role in law enforcement. In the United States and other Western states, critiques of militarism have often targeted police who have been issued weapons, vehicles, and equipment that resemble those of militaries facing battle—because they were quite literally developed for the military. This trend, framed as a benefit to these officers, persists despite evidence that militarized policing reduces trust in law enforcement, doesn't make officers safer, and doesn't reduce violent crime (Mummolo, 2018).

In recent years, attention has centered on police violence while on patrol—especially against Black men—and on the highly militarized responses to protestors. Many people, including children, have been killed in their own homes by highly equipped tactical operations teams who often conduct no-knock raids on homes, sometimes entering the wrong house. Because of the protections afforded to police, loved ones of those killed or harmed in these incidents have little to no recourse. We don't actually know how often this happens, since police departments aren't required to report this information, and because most existing analysis is conducted on incomplete data collected by think tanks or journalists.

Militarization of society can also be seen in how military service is woven into the culture. While the draft ended in the United States in the early 1970s, recruitment campaigns, especially targeting low-income populations, persisted to meet the personnel needs of the world's most dominant military. One in three enlistees is 17 or 18 years old, and militaries often rely on Reserve Officers' Training Corps (ROTC) programs in high schools and colleges to recruit these young adults into the armed forces. Joining the military is presented as just another career alternative. In the early 2000s, legislation like the No Child Left Behind Act even mandated military recruiter access to schools (Hagopian & Barker, 2017).

In many countries, like Russia, China, Sweden, and South Korea, military conscription, usually for males, still exists. In Israel, a country engaged in active, daily conflict, military service is required for almost all citizens above the age of 18, with a few religious, physical, and psychological exceptions. Many who have refused service, usually citing disagreements with the politics of the country or the conflict they are expected to sustain, have been jailed.

In the United States, especially in the post-9/11 period, we were told to fear foreign terrorists and domestic criminals above all other threats, to blindly support our country's military interventions abroad, and to accept any and all domestic restrictions and foreign human rights violations in the name of national security. At the same time, we witnessed the breakdown of many aspects of society that contribute to our own well-being. One study suggested five mechanisms through which militarism negatively impacts global health: diversion of resources, suppression of dissent, military classism, environmental damage, and crime and terrorism (Kiefer, 1992). Even leaving aside the growth of military budgets, a simple look at any sliver of evidence from the past few decades shows just how damaging and all-encompassing militarism can be.

Inequality within countries, a significant contributor to political unrest, has increased significantly. A 2018 report found that the 26 richest people in the world held as much wealth as half of the global population.

Global freedom has been declining for more than a decade, while xenophobia and nationalism are on the upswing. Climate change and environmental destruction are placing unpredictable strains on social, political, and economic dynamics, while technology is increasingly being used to mislead and harm. Women and girls continue to be marginalized while putting in 12.5 billion hours of unpaid work every day—*three times* the hours contributed by the global tech industry (United Nations, 2021a). Ethnic and gender minorities are facing persecution and violence, sometimes encouraged by cynical government actors. Recently, the world experienced a devastating opioid crisis, which in the United States meant a 120% increase in opioid overdose deaths between 2010 and 2018 (WHO, 2021).

Global infrastructure—including railroads, roads, power plants, communications networks, water and sanitation services, and many other facilities and sectors that maintain a functional society—faces regular funding shortfalls. Estimates suggest that investment in global infrastructure needs to be about 20% higher than current allocations to keep up with projected needs by 2050, let alone to modernize energy production, transportation, or any of the other major global sectors (Oxford Economics, 2018). In 2015, around 10% of the population lived on less than $1.90 per day—including one out of five children—and the pandemic could raise the number by 8% (United Nations, 2021b).

Speaking of the COVID-19 pandemic, what better representation of the utter failure of so-called global security, when more than two years into the crisis, we were still struggling to produce enough masks and tests; health care workers began leaving the sector in droves due to burnout; billions remained unvaccinated; and countless lives have been turned upside down through losing a home, losing a job, or losing a loved one.

I could go on and on. Aside from hurting the people directly involved in war, we are hurting ourselves—by investing in war and militarization instead of fulfilling any other part of the social contract. Is this really the future that thousands of years of human development, innovation, and suffering has produced?

REFERENCES

Ahmad, J. (2021). 9/11: how politicians and the media turned terrorism into an Islamic issue. *The Conversation.* https://theconversation.com/9-11-how-politicians-and-the-media-turned-terrorism-into-an-islamic-issue-167733.

Ahmad, M. (2015). The magical realism of body counts: how media credulity and flawed statistics sustain a controversial policy. *Journalism, 17*(1), 18–34.

Al-Oraibi, A., Nellums, L., & Chattopadhyay, K. (2021). COVID-19, conflict, and non-communicable diseases among refugees. *EClinicalMedicine, 34,* 100813. https://doi.org/10.1016/j.eclinm.2021.100813.

Amodu, O. C., Richter, M. S., & Salami, B. O. (2020). A scoping review of the health of conflict-induced internally displaced women in Africa. *International Journal of Environmental Research and Public Health, 17*(4). https://doi.org/10.3390/ijerph17041280.

Awwadawnan, E. (2018, August 2). "I have become lost like my homeland." *Slate.* https://slate.com/news-and-politics/2018/08/one-refugees-firsthand-account-of-his-harrowing-journey-from-syria-to-greece.html.

Barnes, D., Harrison, C., & Heneghan, R. (2004). Health risk and promotion behaviors in refugee populations. *Journal of Health Care for the Poor and Underserved, 15*(3), 347–356.

Bilmes, L. (2021). *The long-term costs of United States care for veterans of the Afghanistan and Iraq Wars.* Costs of War Research Series. https://watson.brown.edu/costsofwar/files/cow/imce/papers/2021/Costs%20of%20War_Bilmes_Long-Term%20Costs%20of%20Care%20for%20Vets_Aug%202021.pdf.

Cantor, D., Swartz, J., Roberts, B., Abbara, A., Ager, A., Bhutta, Z., et al. (2021). Understanding the health needs of internally displaced persons: a scoping review. *Journal of Migration and Health, 4,* 100071. https://doi.org/10.1016/j.jmh.2021.100071.

Cheng, I., Drillich, A., & Schattner, P. (2015). Refugee experiences of general practice in countries of resettlement: a literature review. *British Journal of General Practice, 65*(632), e171–e176. https://doi.org/10.3399/bjgp15X683977.

Cohen, R. (1999). *New challenges for refugee policy: internally displaced persons.* Brookings. https://www.brookings.edu/on-the-record/new-challenges-for-refugee-policy-internally-displaced-persons/.

Copp, T. (2018). DoD: at least 126 bases report water contaminants linked to cancer, birth defects. *MilitaryTimes.* https://www.militarytimes.com/news/your-military/2018/04/26/dod-126-bases-report-water-contaminants-harmful-to-infant-development-tied-to-cancers/.

Costs of War. (2021). *U.S. and allied wounded.* https://watson.brown.edu/costs ofwar/costs/human/military/wounded.

Dator, W., Abunah, H., & Dao-ayen, N. (2018). Health challenges and access to health care among Syrian refugees in Jordan: a review. *Eastern Mediterranean Health Journal, 24*(7), 680–686. https://doi.org/10.26719/2018.24.7.680.

Dye, T. (2007). Contemporary prevalence and prevention of micronutrient deficiencies in refugee settings worldwide. *Journal of Refugee Studies, 20*(1), 108–119.

Enloe, C. (2016). *Globalization and militarism: feminists make the link.* Lanham, MD: Rowman & Littlefield.

Esses, V., Veenvliet, S., Hodson, G., & Mihic, L. (2008). Justice, morality, and the dehumanization of refugees. *Social Justice Research, 21,* 4–25.

Finley, N. (2021, September 14). Virginia and Wisconsin report measles cases among refugees. *AP.* https://apnews.com/article/health-afghanistan-richmond -virginia-taliban-2c7dfd87080c27749d0d36f83b1a74c8.

Gaffney, A., Himmelstein, D., & Woolhandler, S. (2020). *Lack of care for those who serve: health care coverage and access among US veterans, 2019.* (white paper). Public Citizen. https://www.citizen.org/wp-content/uploads/Lack-of-Care-for -those-Who-Serve-Final-DS.pdf?eType=EmailBlastContent&eId=1e9e9344 -4acd-46ca-b7ee-3bf9862d7ed9.

Hagopian, A., & Barker, K. (2016). Countering military recruitment in high schools. In W. Wiist & S. White (Eds.). *Preventing war and promoting peace: a guide for health professionals.* (pp. 230–244). Cambridge: Cambridge University Press.

Haslam, N. (2005). Predisplacement and postdisplacement factors associated with mental health of refugees and internally displaced persons: a meta-analysis. *JAMA, 294*(5), 602–612.

Internal Displacement Monitoring Center (IDMC). (2022). *All-time high of nearly 60 million internally displaced worldwide.* https://www.internal-displacement .org/media-centres/all-time-high-of-nearly-60-million-people-internally -displaced-worldwide.

Kiefer, C. (1992). Militarism and world health. *Social Science and Medicine.* https:// pubmed.ncbi.nlm.nih.gov/1604366/.

Lachmann, R. (2018). These are the VA's 3 main problems—leadership isn't one of them. *The Conversation.* https://theconversation.com/these-are-the-vas-3 -main-problems-leadership-isnt-one-of-them-94220.

Mangrio, E., & Forss, K. (2017). Refugees' experiences of health care in the host country: a scoping review. *BMC Health Services Research, 17.* https://10.1186 /s12913-017-2731-0.

Meadows, S. O., Tanielian, T., & Karney, B. (Eds.). (2016). *How military families respond before, during and after deployment: findings from the RAND Deployment Life Study.* Santa Monica, CA: RAND Corporation. https://www.rand.org/pubs /research_briefs/RB9906.html.

Mummolo, J. (2018). Militarization fails to enhance police safety or reduce crime but may harm police reputation. *PNAS, 115*(37), 9181–9186.

Oxford Economics. (2018). *Global infrastructure outlook.* https://www.oxford economics.com/recent-releases/Global-Infrastructure-Outlook.

Shannon, P., Wieling, E., Simmelink-McCleary, J., & Bechner, E. (2014). Beyond stigma: barriers to discussing mental health in refugee populations. *Journal of Loss and Trauma: International Perspectives on Stress & Coping, 3,* 281–296. https://doi.org/10.1080/15325024.2014.934629.

Shpigel, N. (2020, April 15). Missiles out, ventilators in: Israeli defense contractors answer the coronavirus call. *Haaretz.* https://www.haaretz.com/israel -news/.premium-missiles-to-ventilators-israeli-defense-contractors-answer -the-coronavirus-call-1.8766154.

Syria Relief. (2021). *A place where bad things happen: the public's normalisation of war crimes in Syrian conflict.* https://reliefweb.int/sites/reliefweb.int/files/resources /a%20place%20where%20bad%20things%20happen_report_v6%20%282 %29.pdf.

United Nations (UN). (2019). Responding to the challenges of non-communicable diseases. United Nations Agency Briefs. https://apps.who.int/iris/bitstream /handle/10665/327396/WHO-UNIATF-19.98-eng.pdf.

United Nations (UN). (2021a). *Inequality—bridging the divide.* https://www.un.org /sites/un2.un.org/files/un75_inequality.pdf.

United Nations (UN). (2021b). *Ending poverty.* https://www.un.org/en/global -issues/ending-poverty.

United Nations High Commissioner for Refugees (2021). *Refugee data finder.* https://www.unhcr.org/refugee-statistics/.

USAFacts. (2021). *The veteran population has declined 34% since 2000. Veterans Affairs spending is up 185%.* https://usafacts.org/articles/how-much-money-vet erans-spending-us/.

Woodward, R. (2009). Military geographies. *International Encyclopedia of Human Geography,* 122–127. https://doi.org/10.1016/B978-008044910-4.00712-4.

World Health Organization (WHO). (2021). *Opioid overdose.* https://www.who.int /news-room/fact-sheets/detail/opioid-overdose.

CHAPTER 10

THE BENEFICIARIES OF WAR

What do nations care about the cost of war, if by spending a few hundred millions in steel and gunpowder they can gain a thousand millions in diamonds and cocoa? How can love of humanity appeal as a motive to nations whose love of luxury is built on the inhuman exploitation of human beings, and who, especially in recent years, have been taught to regard these human beings as inhuman?

—W. E. B. DU BOIS, "The African Roots of War" (1915)

Yeah, some folks inherit star-spangled eyes
They send you down to war
And when you ask 'em, "How much should we give?"
They only answer, "More, more, more."

—Creedence Clearwater Revival, "Fortunate Son" (1969)

REMEMBER WHEN GOFUNDME WAS NEW? It seemed like a quirky little site where people who wanted to design an independent video game, take their local band on tour, or write a graphic novel would reach out into the collective good for bits of funding. Today, most of the GoFundMe requests that cross my Twitter feed are desperate requests for money to pay for cancer treatments, funerals for victims of homicide, or classroom supplies. Just the other day, I was disturbed to see video of a "Dash for

Cash" event in South Dakota, where teachers scrambled on an ice hockey rink to grab strewn dollar bills to use for classroom materials. The organizers later apologized for the "degrading" event and donated money to the teachers involved, but that doesn't change the fact that teachers in South Dakota remain among the worst paid in the country (Vigdor, 2021). They are surpassed only by Mississippi, where a teacher with 15 years of experience has an average salary of $46,843 (Sanderlin, 2021). Meanwhile, defense spending makes up nearly half of US annual discretionary spending, which qualifies as either "defense" (military operations, personnel, procurement, and research) or "non-defense," which includes everything else (health, transportation, education, etc.). From the period following 9/11 to 2015, defense spending outpaced non-defense spending every year (CBO, 2021).

I'm not the first, or hundredth, to argue that our priorities as a culture are askew. While much of this book focuses on the United States, many countries around the world feature an unacceptable level of inequality, inconsistent foreign policy decisions, and some level of a militarized culture. War is easier to wage by countries that are wealthy and have enormous power and influence, but political discord is stoked in all countries by people and entities with something to gain. Despite our cultural revulsion for war and its manifestations, war persists. It can't just be that it persists because it is so successful at stopping the bad guys and saving the good guys—that's certainly not the case. Military intervention has occasionally been used for just purposes, and in those cases, civilians are helped. But over and over, the wars we wage end up hurting more people than they help, and we seem to arbitrarily pick and choose which injustices to address. We seem perfectly willing to overlook many genuine cries for help, while throwing endless resources at causes with no discernable achievements and which, in many cases, undermine stated strategic and ethical goals.

If we're going to consider war a public health problem, we need to consider the entirety of the ecosystem in which it operates, in order to know exactly what mitigation measures would be most effective. As with any public health crisis, we must understand how it spreads and

why. Who benefits from perpetuating the paradigm that war is necessary? What are their incentives? Once we see the often unsavory actors
and dynamics that benefit from ongoing war, and recognize how comparatively few civilians are ever actually helped by war, it becomes even
harder to justify.

DEFENSE/ARMS INDUSTRY

Admittedly, the arms industry is an easy one to criticize. Follow the
money, right? The arms industry and its subsidiaries have been the subject of ire from opponents of war and militarization for decades, inspir-
ing countless books, movies, and other media. Indeed, this is the
"military-industrial complex" that outgoing President Dwight Eisenhower warned us about in 1961. A tobacco company benefits when
people smoke, processed food manufacturers benefit when people purchase their foods, and arms manufacturers benefit when people want to
use weapons. The idea of an arms race that simply cannot afford to be
lost—at the expense of just about anything else—has justified trillions of
dollars going towards these industries, which have in turn become a significant driver of jobs in the United States.

With each war, the breadth of governmental power in war-making
(increasingly called "defense") has continued to grow, without ever re-
verting to the pre-war standard. Before World War I, wars were largely
fought, and paid for, as needed. During World War II, factories converted
from civilian to military uses. Unemployment plummeted, as workers
were hired to build the planes, guns, and other equipment needed by the
military. After the war, many factories reverted to pre-war uses as the
economy picked up.

Less than a decade later, however, the Korean War saw a change in
military use, as the Mutual Defense Treaty allowed US troops to stay in
South Korea, developing the norm of a persistent US military presence
around the world. The Korean War also escalated the Cold War, a time
when developing and producing advanced arms were seen as an existential aim. Though the Cold War eventually ended with the dissolution of
the Soviet Union, the world had become permanently more militarized,

and a robust and unquestionable defense budget was now a bipartisan priority for the United States. The defense industry became a staple business, anchoring the economies of many small towns.

Defense production now makes up 10% of manufacturing in the United States, which remains the top global producer of arms, but is also significant to other economies around the world, including China, Russia, and Western Europe (especially France, Germany, Italy, Spain, and the United Kingdom). Many of these countries with large arms industries have at least appeared to prioritize their economic or industrial concerns over strategic ones, although this is hard to determine. This is an industry, after all, and these companies could not survive if wars were still funded on an ad hoc basis. As cynical as it may sound, war is a business.

And for now, at least, business is booming: in 2019 alone, the top five arms companies (all US-based) registered $166 billion in sales. Overall, arms sales increased by 8.5% between 2018 and 2019 (SIPRI, 2020). Arms exports accounted for $175 billion in sales for the United States in 2020, which the Department of Defense (DoD) claims is "strengthening U.S. Alliances and attracting new international partners, and adding thousands of jobs to the U.S. economy and sustaining many thousands more" (DoD, 2020). How can one not support an industry that creates so many jobs? This is the catch-22 we've created.

Yet many well-documented human rights abuses have been committed with these very weapons, such as by Saudi Arabia against Yemen. Prior to the current war, US arms sales to Saudi Arabia were about $3 billion over several years; between 2015 and 2020, that number skyrocketed to $64 billion, despite multiple accounts of Saudi forces bombing civilian targets and a Saudi blockade on Yemen that has contributed to near-famine conditions (Riedel, 2021). Many have called on the United States to end these sales, but the US has been slow to take any meaningful action on this issue, whether under Republican or Democratic administrations.

The United States has in fact sold arms to *both sides* of multiple conflicts, and because weapons are easily stolen or otherwise misplaced, US soldiers have sometimes faced enemy forces armed with US weapons. The case for arms sales as beneficial to either long-term global security or domestic economics does not have much evidence behind it; yet exploring alternatives on either front is seen by many policymakers as not sufficiently pragmatic. If anything, our arms sales make global tensions more likely, as nations witness their antagonistic neighbors building up weapons or troops.

From 2001 to 2011, the DoD spent approximately $46 billion on projects that failed, including the development of new satellite systems and helicopters. Most of the successful programs of that period involved simply modifying preexisting systems, leading one analysis to report that "a significant portion of DoD's investment in modernization over the past decade did not result in force modernization" (Harrison, 2011). At the same time, soldiers were paying up to $900 for their own helmets and even medical supplies (Tritten, 2016).

Yes, failure is a part of innovation; and yes, there were likely some useful discoveries made in working on those systems prior to their failure. But the notion that military equipment must consistently be getting better—and that this can happen only as a result of spending billions on brand-new technologies that are announced with much fanfare but that fail much more quietly—is dangerous. Arms sales to nations that violate human rights are rarely questioned, due in part to the United States' economic dependence on the arms industry, but also due to the ongoing fiction that selling arms to these countries somehow gives the United States more sway in these nations' political decisions. Arms sales are also seen as indicators of strength and political support.

At the same time, the military often does not know where its stockpiles are; the only goods that are consistently tracked are nuclear weapons, and even those have sometimes been accidentally shipped to the wrong location or otherwise misplaced. Yet the Pentagon bristles at meaningful investigations and inquiries into its spending and functioning, claiming they are either classified security issues or else too complex for outsiders to understand (Taibbi, 2019). Few industries are allowed to fail so expensively, with such little accountability, and yet with no question that the next new idea will be fully funded. The ongoing wars justify the new ideas, and the new ideas make it easier and less painful—for rich and powerful countries—to keep the wars going.

POLITICAL STAKEHOLDERS

The arms industry wouldn't be nearly so powerful without the politicians that advocate for it and give it such leeway, while exercising poor congressional and executive oversight of the Pentagon. Many politicians (along with political parties and other stakeholders) are economically or rhetorically dependent on supporting a robust military and arms industry, and they get a lot of help in staying that way. In 2020 alone, five of the top US defense contractors spent $60 million on lobbying, while in the past 20 years, defense-related lobbyists and donors directed $285 million towards political campaigns, and another $2.5 billion towards lobbying (Auble, 2021).

Many of these lobbyists are former government officials, but many current government officials have ties to the defense industry as well. For example, General Lloyd Austin, who retired from the armed services in 2016, quickly joined the board of Raytheon Technologies, where he sat until his nomination as the US secretary of defense in 2021. In 2020, 51 members of Congress or their spouses owned between $2.3 and $5.8 million in defense contractor stocks, which they are not required to divest from, despite their role in national security and their knowledge of foreign operations that are beneficial to defense stocks (Shaw & Moore, 2020).

Defense contractors also remain significant players in the approximately 15 states where they primarily operate, including the largest in the country (e.g., Texas, California, Florida, and Pennsylvania). Many representatives from these states actively cater to the policy needs of these industries. Interestingly, even in Europe, where all types of sectors are highly regulated, the arms industry is comparatively much less so, indicating the political potency of the issue (TNI, 2020). When the item being manufactured is not useful in day-to-day life, it seems more than plausible that policy decisions on warfare may be driven at least partly by justifying the existence of these economically beneficial defense manufacturers, whether for personal or community profit.

Aside from the economic benefits, politicians pick up significant political and social capital in certain audiences for being seen as "hawkish," meaning they are quicker to suggest war as a solution to a foreign policy problem. While this can be found in pockets in democratic societies, "hawkishness" can be an entire organizing premise for authoritarians or those who support them. Authoritarianism relies on conformity, obedience, and—importantly—out-group aggression. Authoritarian leaders rile up their supporters with fear and with the promise that they will be aggressive towards those that threaten the in-group, at all costs. Force is the currency of authoritarianism, and the promise of potentially using that force has propelled authoritarian-leaning politicians to the helms of governments around the world. Even in democratic states, perceived external threats can push societies to accept authoritarian policies, including censorship, surveillance, torture, and preemptive war, as was seen among Americans post-9/11 (Hetherington & Suhay, 2011).

Meanwhile, being hesitant to engage in war is framed as unrealistic, dangerous, and potentially even treasonous. In 2001, Congresswoman Barbara Lee of California cast the one and only vote in the entire US Congress against the war in Afghanistan. Giving a speech on the House floor, Lee pleaded, "However difficult this vote may be, some of us must urge the use of restraint. Our country is in a state of mourning. Some of us must say, 'Let's step back for a moment, let's just pause, just for a minute, and think through the implications of our actions today, so that this does not spiral out of control.'" Members of the press called her a "clueless liberal" and a "supporter of America's enemies." Her office received death threats, often tinged with racism and sexism, and she went on to defend her position in the press for weeks. She also consistently introduced legislation to repeal the authorization, which finally passed the House—but not the Senate—in 2019 (Brockell, 2021). Today, after trillions of dollars spent and thousands of lives lost in Afghanistan with little sustainable progress to show for it, together with exponentially declining public support and a "War on Terror" that has spiraled out of control, the wisdom of her words and vote seems apparent.

Evidence shows that how politicians talk about matters of war and foreign policy matters, as it shapes the opinions of the public, who have less information and are less engaged in the minutiae of such issues

(Berinsky, 2007). Yet the drumbeat of war persists, now most loudly against Iran and China, through some of the same voices that supported the disastrous wars in Iraq and Afghanistan. Unlike Barbara Lee, these politicians were rarely if ever expected to justify their viewpoint or to reflect on the folly of their decisions, and to this day many of them remain widely called upon for their foreign policy analysis on cable news shows and in op-eds in prestigious newspapers. The lesson learned by politicians is that it's better to call for war and be wrong—blame the press, blame the people of the country you invaded, blame the intelligence community, blame the president—than to call for peace, introspection, or even a robust debate. Do you love your country? If so, it seems the way to prove it is to support going to war at every opportunity.

The Department of Defense, which was called the Department of War until 1947, is often funded with even more money than it requests. It is well known for being bloated and complex, but it frames these flaws not as points for improvement but as justification for more funding and less oversight. A 2015 study found that streamlining the Pentagon would save $125 billion. To put this into context: the entire budget of the United States Centers for Disease Control and Prevention (CDC) for 2020, the year the worst pandemic in a century entered our lives, was just above $6.5 billion (CDC, 2020). At the time, Democratic Senator Bernie Sanders noted, "It is time to fundamentally change our national priorities. In the midst of the worst public health crisis in over 100 years and the most severe economic downturn since the Great Depression, we do not need to authorize $740.5 billion in bombs, weapons, fighter jets and endless wars." (They did.)

The Pentagon is still handsomely funded after failed audits on top of failed wars, and has been endlessly supported in a "dominance over deterrence" strategy. The thing is, dominance has no ceiling: as your perceived opponents build up their militaries and weaponry, you must keep going as well (Hester, 2021). What *can't* be justified under such a paradigm? Even police departments across the United States have been equipped with $1.6 billion in goods from the Pentagon since 9/11, including armored vehicles being used in American neighborhoods. This also informs how politicians view defense spending—if you question or limit spending, you are seen as actively undercutting the US position of dominance.

RACISTS

Is everything about race these days? No, but most aspects of our lives are racialized, and war is no exception. The United Nations recognizes that "racism continues to be a major obstacle to friendly and peaceful relations among peoples and nations" (2012). It has been used, both implicitly and explicitly, to justify endless acts of cruelty throughout history, including but not limited to the Holocaust, internment of Japanese Americans, Japanese war crimes against the Chinese, chattel slavery in the United States and elsewhere, European colonial violence against natives, maltreatment of refugees, and apartheid in South Africa. While there remains a conspicuous lack of studies connecting racism to war, we would be remiss not to consider this pervasive social force—which in recent decades has shaped issues as varied as housing, health care, public transportation, criminal justice, and the environment—as one of the core elements driving the most organized forms of violence, up to and including war.

It should be no surprise that racists love war: it provides an outlet for racial resentments and vengeance, helps to easily identify an "other," and builds solidarity among the in-group. Racism provides cover for the belief in "just oppression," defined as "a racist belief in domination and compliance, to take it for granted that something like human dignity no longer matters, and therefore we can overlook abuse, violence, and destruction by blaming the 'other'" (Batur, 2007, p. 444). Racism is the entire driving force behind acts of war like genocide, ethnic cleansing, and forms of collective punishment. The victim does not need to be guilty of any specific act themselves; they are guilty as a result of their identity and associations.

Racism is useful in dehumanizing an enemy and justifying attacks and horrific acts against them. It enables leaders to invoke racist tropes and threaten violence to cover for lack of ideas or consistent values. Racists see their own physical violence as valiant, while painting their victims, if they retaliate, as inherently violent barbarians. They enact racist policies under the guise of security or bureaucracy as a form of structural violence. Racism provides justification for causes that aren't actually based on anything substantial. Indeed, the effects of racism are insidious in all aspects of war and militarization; evidence shows that in situations of tension with other countries, white Americans with racist beliefs are more in favor of military action against those countries whose residents are nonwhite, for example China and Iran (Medenica & Ebner, 2021).

But racism doesn't just affect political conflict abroad. Racism is found within the US military, including individual discriminatory incidents and the activity of white supremacist cells (Stafford, Laporta, & Morrison, 2021). A 2017 survey of American service members found that 31% of Black troops reported racial discrimination or harassment in just the previous year (along with 23% of Asian American and 21% of Hispanic troops) (Coughlin, 2021). Racism also changes how we view our fellow citizen in times of war; consider that 93% of Americans supported the internment of Japanese immigrants during World War II, 59% supported the internment of Japanese American citizens, and the US Supreme Court upheld restrictions on Japanese Americans at least 12 times (USHMM, 2021). After the 9/11 attacks, hate crimes against those perceived as Muslim or Arab skyrocketed. One man, upon being arrested for the murder of a Sikh man he perceived as one of "the ragheads responsible for September 11," told police, "I stand for America all the way! I'm an American. Go ahead. Arrest me and let those terrorists run wild!" (HRW, 2002).

Much of the "counter-terrorism" initiatives during the Global War on Terror in countries like the United States and the United Kingdom seemed entirely based on anti-Muslim racism, and this did not go unnoticed by the public. In 2002, a year after 9/11, 32% of Republicans in the United States thought that Islam was more likely than other religions to encourage violence. After decades of rhetoric from primarily Republican politicians and media figures painting Islam as a threat, today fully 72% of Republicans express this view (Democrats went from 23% to 32% in that same time period) (Hartig & Doherty, 2021).

Aside from overstating the threat posed by external racialized groups, racism contributes to one of the most significant threats faced by people in developed countries. Ethno-nationalist and white supremacist movements are gaining ground across the United States and Europe. The white supremacist who killed 50 people at two mosques in New Zealand in 2019 decried immigration as "the complete racial and cultural replacement of the European people." Far-right-wing violence has killed more Americans than Jihadists have in the years since 9/11; Attorney General Merrick Garland specified that the greatest domestic threat at the moment stems from "those who advocate for the superiority of the white race" (Sullivan & Benner, 2021).

Indeed, it was largely these anti-government and white supremacist forces who perpetuated the attack on the US Capitol on January 6, 2021. Significantly, more than 20 of those arrested in the attack had ties to the US military. If the perpetrators had been of any other race, this event would likely have precipitated serious discussion of political or even military intervention. It is worth considering why it has not.

MEDIA

On September 8, 2002, Judith Miller published the article that contributed to the end of her storied career as a journalist at the *New York Times*. In her article, "Threats and Responses: The Iraqis; U.S. Says Hussein Intensifies Quest for A-Bomb Parts," Miller and her co-author Michael R. Gordon cited several pieces of purported evidence, primarily from anonymous American officials and Iraqi defectors, that Iraq was in serious pursuit of nuclear weapons, potentially even on the way to using biological and chemical weapons. In one memorable quote regarding potential military intervention, a Bush administration official said, "The question is not, why now? The question is why waiting is better. The closer Saddam Hussein gets to a nuclear weapon, the harder he will be to deal with." The Bush administration then cited the article as evidence in their own prelude to war.

Miller went on to write several unsubstantiated stories about weapons of mass destruction in Iraq (weapons we now know never existed) and won a Pulitzer Prize for her writing on global terror post-9/11. While almost all journalists and guests on cable news shows held a pro-war stance at the time, once it came to light that much of Miller's reporting was based on faulty information and discredited sources, her credibility was ruined, and she left the *Times* (Seelye, 2005). A decade later, when she was on a book tour, TV host Jon Stewart articulated the belief of many about the impact of her work: "I believe that you helped the administration take us to the most devastating mistake in foreign policy that we've made in 100 years." In her response, she defended herself and her reporting by asserting, "All journalists are manipulated and all politicians lie" (Emery, 2015).

"If it bleeds, it leads" is a trope of journalism, and especially of cable television news, perhaps first popularized by a 1989 article by Eric Poole for *New York* magazine. The piece, which focused on local news stations and how they cover crime and violence, critiqued the "show biz" nature of news and how delicate human issues are treated as entertainment. Poole observed, "The thoughtful report is buried because sensational stories must launch the broadcast: If it bleeds, it leads." However, this isn't necessarily always the case with war. In fact, during the 1991 Gulf War, the military instated a policy barring media coverage of the flag-draped coffins of American servicepeople killed in action. Although they claimed it was to protect the privacy of service members' families, many critics argued it was to prevent the American public from understanding the true cost of war. But the media doesn't need photos of coffins or grieving families to portray the costs of war—as I've attempted to illustrate throughout this book, there is copious evidence of its folly. Instead, the media often seems to prefer publishing feel-good stories about soldiers returning home, or the latest despicable antics of terrorists. These are the types of stories that sell the fallacy that war isn't so bad, and even that war really is necessary. Who needs context, history, critique, or data, when we can instead watch a moving segment on how happy this soldier's adorable dog is to have him home?

Likewise, the media is not particularly adept at explaining international humanitarian laws and norms to their audience, or how and why certain actors are violating them. They are less skeptical of official government sources and press releases than evidence suggests they should be, and their use of language, framing, and perspective plays a significant role in who is seen as a victim or perpetrator. News anchors openly pontificate about issues on which neither they nor their guests are experts, and miss opportunities to ask challenging or probing questions when they do bring experts or government officials onto their programs. This is not an issue unique to the American press—the German press faced significant criticism for being too susceptible to misinformation fed to them by political and military sources during the Gulf War and the war in Kosovo (Eilders, 2005).

It is not necessarily that individual journalists want war—although some certainly argue for it regularly—but that many journalists depend on access to high-ranking government officials and do not want to threaten that access by presenting critical coverage. Independent media outlets are often more critical and overtly anti-war, as well as more likely to include marginalized voices, but may not have the reach or prestige of more mainstream outlets that prioritize access and the image of rigid neutrality—leading them to present "both sides" of issues that ethically, morally, and legally don't really have two equally justifiable viewpoints.

Further, the viewpoints of "both sides" are often voiced by pundits or powerful figures, often situated in the West, rather than by the people on the ground actually affected by the events, who are frequently considered too biased or involved to be trusted to describe their own lived experience. For example, the *New York Times* has been among the top legacy publications for decades, documenting countless political crises and shaping how millions of people not just receive but interpret the news. Between 1970 and 2019, the paper published 2,490 op-ed pieces on Israel/Palestine. Only 46 were written by Palestinians—less than 2% (Nassar, 2020). During the withdrawal of American troops from Afghanistan, which blanketed American media for weeks, less than one-third (31%) of sources on the three major cable news networks—ABC, CBS, and NBC—were Afghan. Despite the attention paid to the potential plight of Afghan women under a restrictive Taliban regime, they made up only 5% of guests (FAIR, 2022).

Then there is overt manipulation of the content offered to viewers. During the Iraq war, ratings for Fox News skyrocketed. The tenor of the channel was straightforward: full support for President Bush and the war. American flags and troop montages. Iraqis? They're "terror goons" and "the great unwashed." The UN was "dopey," and those who didn't support the war were "sickening." CNN, CBS, and MSNBC all saw some ratings increases for their war coverage, but they trailed Fox. In an effort to be more welcoming to viewers, MSNBC, whose hosts at the time were largely against the war, fired some of its commentators and replaced them with more conservative, pro-war voices (Rutenberg, 2003).

Corporate media is, ultimately, a business. A media business relies on the number of viewers, not strategic or cogent viewpoints. Especially when it comes to issues of foreign policy—as many media outlets are cutting international correspondents—media coverage tends to be racialized, elitist, uncritical, and sporadic. Coverage about war usually does not become negative or critical until elites start to critique the war, or events on the ground are too devastating to ignore (Aday, 2018). Many large media outlets are so cautious about being perceived as having any hint of political bias, and determined at all costs to cover every issue as though all viewpoints are equally valid, that they miss the bias that is truly damaging to societies: the bias towards stories that are entertaining, sensational, and trendy over those that expose and critique the structures and systems that govern our lives (Hershey, 2020).

Then there is the fact that many media corporations today are just one cog in a larger corporate machine—a machine that likely doesn't appreciate coverage that criticizes the very systems that benefit its owners, associated policymakers, and other powerful players in and around the industry. Indeed, it is estimated that 90% of American media now is controlled by about six companies. This concentration of media ownership limits diversity of opinion, especially regarding critical viewpoints, and instead pushes media to shape the culture around the preferred narratives of media owners (Uzuegbunam, 2020).

But it does not, unfortunately, end with economic incentives. The media cannot start wars, but it can fan the social dynamics that contribute to war. The media plays a significant role in shaping public opinion by (for instance) whom they choose to feature, how they choose to question them, what topics they cover, and how critically they cover them. During the Rwandan genocide, local news and radio stations in that country spread propaganda and helped mobilize citizens towards hatred and violence. Several Rwandan journalists were even found guilty of inciting genocide.

Then there is "yellow journalism," a crude term for news that prioritizes sensationalism over reality. This propaganda-like form of media has certainly helped provoke wars before. In fact, the term is most associated with the coverage of the Spanish-American War in the late 1800s. A US battleship named the *Maine* sank near Cuba, and without evidence, publishers blamed the Spanish and escalated the anti-Spanish rhetoric that had been selling papers for years. "Remember the Maine!" became the rallying cry for war, and papers would outright fabricate stories to feed the public outcry for vengeance. When one photographer based in Cuba sent word to his paper's publisher in the United States that there was no war to cover, the publisher reportedly told him, "You furnish the pictures. I'll furnish the war." While the *Maine* was not the only reason for the war, it played a large part in its inception (PBS, 1999). Furnish the war, indeed.

REFERENCES

Aday, S. (2018). The US media, foreign policy, and public support for War. In K. Kenski & K. Jamieson (Eds.). *The Oxford Handbook of Political Communication.* Oxford: Oxford University Press.

Auble, D. (2021). Capitalizing on conflict: how defense contractors and foreign nations lobby for arms sales. *Open Secrets.* https://www.opensecrets.org/news /reports/capitalizing-on-conflict.

Batur, P. (2007). Heart of violence: global racism, war, and genocide. In H. Vera & J. R. Feagin (Eds.). *Handbook of the sociology of racial and ethnic relations.* Boston: Springer. https://doi.org/10.1007/978-0-387-70845-4_22.

Berinsky, A. (2007). Assuming the costs of war: events, elites, and American public support for military conflict. *Journal of Politics, 69*(4), 975–997.

Brockell, G. (2021, August 17). She was the only member of Congress to vote against war in Afghanistan. Some called her a traitor. *The Washington Post.* https://www .washingtonpost.com/history/2021/08/17/barbara-lee-afghanistan-vote/.

Centers for Disease Control and Prevention (CDC). (2020). *CDC—budget request overview.* https://www.cdc.gov/budget/documents/fy2020/cdc-overview-fact sheet.pdf.

Congressional Budget Office (CBO). (2021). *The federal budget in fiscal year 2020: a closer look at discretionary spending.* https://www.cbo.gov/system/files/2021 -04/57172-discretionary-spending.pdf.

Coughlin, S. (2021). Racism and discrimination in the military and the health of US service members. *Military Medicine, 186*(5–6).

Department of Defense (DoD). (2020). *FY2020 security cooperation numbers.* Security Cooperation Agency. https://www.dsca.mil/news-media/news-archive/fy2020-security-cooperation-numbers.

Du Bois, W. (1915). The African roots of war. *The Atlantic.* https://www.theatlantic.com/magazine/archive/1915/05/the-african-roots-of-war/528897/.

Eilders, C. (2005). Media under fire: fact and fiction in conditions of war. *International Review of the Red Cross, 87*(860), 639–648.

Emery, D. (2015). Jon Stewart rips apart Judith Miller over Iraq reporting: you pushed us into "devastating" mistake. *The Wrap.* https://www.thewrap.com/jon-stewart-rips-apart-judith-miller-over-iraq-reporting-you-pushed-us-into-devastating-mistake/.

Fairness & Accuracy in Reporting (FAIR). (2022). *Media literacy guide: how to detect bias in news media.* https://fair.org/take-action-now/media-activism-kit/how-to-detect-bias-in-news-media/.

Gordon, M., & Miller, J. (2002). Threats and responses: the Iraqis; U.S. says Hussein intensifies quest for A-bomb parts. *The New York Times.* https://www.nytimes.com/2002/09/08/world/threats-responses-iraqis-us-says-hussein-intensifies-quest-for-bomb-parts.html.

Harrison, T. (2011). Analysis of the FY 2012 defense budget. *CSBA.* https://csbaonline.org/uploads/documents/2011.07.16-FY-2012-Defense-Budget.pdf.

Hartig, H., & Doherty, C. (2021). *Two decades later, the enduring legacy of 9/11.* Pew Research Center. https://www.pewresearch.org/politics/2021/09/02/two-decades-later-the-enduring-legacy-of-9-11/.

Hershey, M. (2020). Political bias in media doesn't threaten democracy—other, less visible biases do. *The Conversation.* https://theconversation.com/political-bias-in-media-doesnt-threaten-democracy-other-less-visible-biases-do-144844.

Hester, A. (2021). Why Congress keeps giving the Pentagon more money than it needs. *Responsible Statecraft.* https://responsiblestatecraft.org/2021/08/03/why-congress-keeps-giving-the-pentagon-more-money-than-it-needs/.

Hetherington, M., & Suhay, E. (2011). Authoritarianism, threat, and Americans' support for the War on Terror. *American Journal of Political Science, 55*(3), 546–560.

Human Rights Watch (HRW). (2002). *"WE ARE NOT THE ENEMY": Hate crimes against Arabs, Muslims, and those perceived to be Arab or Muslim after September 11.* https://www.hrw.org/reports/2002/usahate/index.htm#TopOfPage.

Medenica, V., & Ebner, D. (2021). Racial bias makes white Americans more likely to support wars in nonwhite foreign countries—new study. *The Conversation.* https://theconversation.com/racial-bias-makes-white-americans-more-likely-to-support-wars-in-nonwhite-foreign-countries-new-study-157638.

Nassar, M. (2020). US media talks a lot about Palestinians—just without Palestinians. +972 *Magazine.* https://www.972mag.com/us-media-palestinians/.

PBS. (1999). *Yellow journalism.* https://www.pbs.org/crucible/bio_hearst.html.

Poole, E. (1989, October 9). Grins, gore, and videotape: the trouble with local TV news. *New York Magazine.*

Riedel, B. (2021). *It's time to stop US arms sales to Saudi Arabia.* Brookings. https://www.brookings.edu/blog/order-from-chaos/2021/02/04/its-time-to-stop-us-arms-sales-to-saudi-arabia/.

Rutenberg, J. (2003, April 16). A nation at war: the news media; cable's war coverage suggests a new "Fox Effect" on television journalism. *The New York Times.* https://www.nytimes.com/2003/04/16/us/nation-war-media-cable-s-war-coverage-suggests-new-fox-effect-television.html.

Sanderlin, L. (2021, September 15). Experts: Mississippi teacher pay needs to increase if state wants to keep its educators. *Clarion Ledger.* https://www.clarionledger.com/story/news/politics/2021/09/16/mississippi-senate-holds-hearings-teacher-pay-health-benefits/8347223002/.

Seelye, K. (2005, November 10). Times reporter agrees to leave the paper. *The New York Times.* https://www.nytimes.com/2005/11/10/business/media/times-reporter-agrees-to-leave-the-paper.html.

Shaw, D., & Moore, D. (2020). The members of Congress who profit from war. *The American Prospect.* https://prospect.org/power/the-members-of-congress-who-profit-from-war/.

Stockholm International Peace Research Institute (SIPRI). (2020). *Global arms industry: sales by the top 25 companies up 8.5 per cent; Big players active in Global South.* https://www.sipri.org/media/press-release/2020/global-arms-industry-sales-top-25-companies-85-cent-big-players-active-global-south.

Stafford, K., Laporta, J., & Morrison, A. (2021). AP report: deep-rooted racism and discrimination permeate US military. *Associated Press.* https://www.pbs.org/newshour/nation/ap-report-deep-rooted-racism-and-discrimination-permeate-u-s-military.

Sullivan, E., & Benner, K. (2021). Top law enforcement officials say the biggest domestic terror threat comes from white supremacists. *The New York Times.* https://www.nytimes.com/2021/05/12/us/politics/domestic-terror-white-supremacists.html.

Taibbi, M. (2019). The Pentagon's bottomless money pit. *Rolling Stone.* https://
www.rollingstone.com/politics/politics-features/pentagon-budget-mystery
-807276/amp/?_twitter_impression=true.

Transnational Institute (TNI). (2021). *Smoking guns.* https://www.tni.org/en
/publication/smoking-guns.

Tritten, T. (2016, February 25). Lacking basic gear, special operators stuck buying their own equipment. *Stars and Stripes.* https://www.stripes.com/news
/lacking-basic-gear-special-operators-stuck-buying-their-own-equipment-1
.396109.

United Nations (UN). (2012). United Nations experts say racism is still igniting
and fuelling violence and conflict. *ReliefWeb.* https://reliefweb.int/report/world
/united-nations-experts-say-racism-still-igniting-and-fuelling-violence-and
-conflict.

United States Holocaust Memorial Museum (USHMM). (2021). Public opinion
poll on Japanese internment. *Americans and the Holocaust.* https://exhibi
tions.ushmm.org/americans-and-the-holocaust/main/japanese-american
-internment.

Uzuegbunam, C. (2020). Concentration of media ownership. *The SAGE International Encyclopedia of Mass Media and Society.* https://doi.org/10.4135
/9781483375519.

Vigdor, N. (2021, December 13). Hockey team apologizes for "degrading" cash
grab for teachers. *The New York Times.* https://www.nytimes.com/2021/12/13
/us/south-dakota-teachers-dash-for-cash.html.

CHAPTER 11

THE HUMANITARIAN RESPONSE TO WAR

Not all the investment for Europe's progress came from the sweated labour of European workers and farmers. It came also from the people of Asia, Africa, and South America who were denied a fair return for their work and their produce. Empires have ended, but the colonial pattern of economy remains with us in one form or another . . . Aid is only partial recompense for what the superior economic power of the advanced countries denies us through trade.

—INDIRA GANDHI,
prime minister of India, addressing the UN General Assembly Plenary Meeting (1968)

I pulled up behind a Cadillac
We were waiting for the light
And I took a look at his license plate
It said, "just ice"
Is justice just ice?
Governed by greed and lust?
Just the strong doing what they can
And the weak suffering what they must?

—JONI MITCHELL, "Sex Kills" (1994)

AS I FIRST SAT DOWN to write this chapter, the third major variant of the COVID-19 pandemic (Omicron) was raging throughout the world.

Back in March 2020, we were told it would be a few weeks of lockdown. Years in, however, COVID-19 has led to nearly seven million confirmed global deaths and likely many more due to underdiagnosis. We have gone through various stages of lockdowns and other significant life disruptions and delays. And today, epidemiologists are telling us that the window to completely eradicate COVID-19 has closed—that we'll probably have to live with some form of the virus forever. Pandemic fatigue seems like an understatement at this point. But the vaccines were developed at a record pace—how are we still in this mess?

Well, according to many medical professionals, epidemiologists, social scientists, and ethicists, one of the biggest problems was vaccine inequity. Sure, the vaccines were developed quickly, but only a few manufacturers could make them, and wealthy countries bought up millions of doses immediately. The underlying assumption was that once an individual was vaccinated, their life could resume as normal. And this was the case—for a few months. Summer 2021 brought a brief sense of normalcy for a tiny fraction of the world's population. But then the Delta variant emerged, first identified in India, where only a small percentage of the population had even received a first dose of a vaccine. Instead of expediting vaccine manufacturing for global distribution, wealthy nations began administering boosters and vaccinating children before high-risk people and health care workers in many countries had been vaccinated at all. That worked too—for a few more months.

Then the Omicron variant, much more contagious than its predecessors, was identified in South Africa. The message was clear: the more we allow this virus to proliferate around the world, the higher potential for variants that evade preexisting vaccines and protective measures. But, again, instead of instituting vaccine waivers, ensuring adequate global personal protective equipment supply, and accelerating equitable distribution of existing vaccines, wealthy countries started considering a fourth booster dose and temporarily banned flights from Africa. By the end of 2021, only 8.3% of people in low-income countries had received a first vaccination dose. In light of increasing variants and unmet vaccine donation commitments, Dr. Tedros Adhanom Ghebreyesus, director-general of the WHO, said vaccine equity was "not rocket science, nor charity. It is smart public health and in everyone's best interest" (United Nations, 2021c).

Charity is an interesting concept to consider in light of a devastating global pandemic. Is it charity to ensure populations with poor health systems have access to equipment and medications that not only save lives but prevent further proliferation and mutation of a disease that has killed millions and disrupted the lives of billions? It sounds more like common sense, but charity was exactly how it was treated. While the United States and other wealthy nations have pledged to donate billions of vaccines in the coming years, it's not close to sufficient nor fast enough. Many of the doses donated so far arrived close to their expiration date, or the country they were sent to did not have sufficient capacity to store or distribute the inconsistent shipments of vaccines. Meanwhile, these same wealthy countries threw away millions of expired doses they had purchased but had no demand for, and many more precious vaccines were otherwise ruined or corrupted. This certainly doesn't seem like charity—yet the same limitations that have stymied the global COVID-19 vaccine effort play out in the world's most fragile environments every day.

There are approximately 570,000 humanitarian aid workers in the world who work in thousands of agencies. Some are huge, like those associated with the United Nations (the World Food Programme, the UN High Commissioner for Refugees, and the UN Children's Fund [UNICEF] are the three biggest spenders). As a whole, the UN humanitarian agencies spend about as much as all other nongovernmental organizations (NGOs) combined, but much of the UN's money goes to smaller NGOs in the form of grants (Clarke, 2018). Other significant players in conflict-affected areas include Médecins Sans Frontières, the International Federation of Red Cross and Red Crescent Societies, Oxfam International, Mercy Corps, and Save the Children. Additionally, there are thousands of small- and medium-sized grassroots NGOs that are based in-country and made up primarily of local staff who often risk their lives for little pay.

Aid can come in the form of assistance, goods, and, much more rarely, cash. Different types of aid have different purposes: humanitarian assistance meant to provide urgent interventions in areas of acute crisis; assistance for social, economic, and political development; and security assistance, like providing weapons, training, or other military support to allies. Aside from security assistance, most aid funding doesn't actually go to governments themselves because fragile states may not have the means, capacity, or desire to implement needed programs. Instead, it is funneled to large and small NGOs, especially in areas of service delivery. Although most Americans believe foreign aid takes up a quarter of the federal budget, in reality it's less than 1% (Ingram, 2019). No country, in fact, contributes more than 1% of their budget to aid.

If war is a public health crisis, then what is the medicine? Decades of evidence suggest that humanitarian aid, often proposed as the main solution to meeting the needs of conflict-affected populations, has many benefits and has certainly made contributions to increasing life expectancy, decreasing poverty, and preventing the spread of diseases like smallpox, polio, and HIV. But humanitarian aid cannot replace functional institutions or a robust social contract between a government and a resident. The recent example of COVID-19 vaccine inequity demonstrates the risks of depending on humanitarian aid to meet crucial societal needs. Further, there is the reality that humanitarian aid is a system made up of people, and people are flawed. Dozens of accusations of corruption, abuse, and discrimination have been made against some of the most credible and respected aid agencies in the world, yet affected citizens have little avenue for recourse. Combine these bad actors, even if just a few, with access to marginalized populations who have little agency, and very unfortunate outcomes can occur that can erode hard-won trust gained with populations who have little trust left to offer.

It's tough to make a critical argument about humanitarian aid—what could possibly be bad about giving food to hungry people or medical care to those without? We cannot overlook the good that humanitarian aid has done or the genuinely good intentions of many people who work in the aid industry. The purpose of aid is not, and never has been, to end war, so we can't blame it for not doing so. But even as a tool for promoting sustainable or meaningful development, aid has a track record that is mixed at best. Optimistically, it is a bandage, offering some protection to the vulnerable while the wound heals. Today's wars, however, don't end quickly or cleanly. Many aid operations are expected to continue for many years as other conflicts or disasters continue to occur. It is clear that humanitarian aid does play a role in supporting fragile populations, but are we expecting it to do too much—or too little?

IT'S NOT ENOUGH

The war in Syria is identified as one of the worst crises of our time. More than 14 million people currently require humanitarian aid. The United States is by far the biggest funder of aid to Syria, contributing about a third of total aid on an annual basis. This amounts to about $12 billion since the war started in 2012. Countries like Germany and the United Kingdom contribute millions more. Yet in just the past year, an additional 4.5 million Syrians were made food insecure, adding to the almost 8 million from the year before. That equates to about 60% of the population. For many, food from the World Food Programme (WFP) may be their only source of sustenance. "The situation has never been worse," the WFP Country Director in Syria said in 2021, years after the peak of the bombardment campaigns (United Nations, 2021a). Half of Syrian children are malnourished, and 2.5 million children are out of school. Almost the entire Syrian population—90%—live in poverty. Only 58% of the country's hospitals are functional (United Nations, 2021b). We can understand that such a complex emergency might not be getting better, but how can it be getting so drastically worse, especially when the worst of the physical violence seems to have ended?

In 2019, global humanitarian aid stood at about $29.6 billion. While a significant amount of money, this number represented the first time aid funding had dropped since 2012—a 5% reduction from 2018. Of the 36 appeals for aid coordinated by the United Nations in 2019, only nine received more than 75% of the requested funds. A third received less than half of what was requested, while the Democratic Republic of the Congo received less than 25%. Syria and Yemen alone account for about a third of aid appeals, but Syria only received 58% of the requested funds. Overall, total funding shortfalls were about $11.1 billion; only 64% of what was requested was ultimately delivered. Although this seems low, it was the second-highest percentage of met aid requests in the past decade (Development Initiatives, 2020). To put this into perspective, the cost of the 2016 Summer Olympic Games in Brazil was $20 billion, while the 2018 Winter Games in South Korea had a price tag of $13 billion. While this, of course, isn't a one-to-one comparison, what we can quickly realize is that the money exists to fully fund these aid appeals and then some; we, as a society, just choose not to, often citing economic limitations when the reality seems to be more political (more on that in a bit).

The money provided often fills urgent gaps in care and undoubtedly prevents widespread famine and other crises, but the extent to which it gives people genuine stability is limited. A recent survey of aid recipients found that only 26% said that the aid mostly or completely met their needs. Most have to supplement the aid with work (if employment is even available or safe), remittances, or savings if they are able (OECD, 2019). Further, aid rarely meets other financial needs of fragile populations, like addressing personal debt, that exacerbate poverty. It also seldom comes in the form of unconditional cash that allows recipients to spend money where they deem it as most needed. Thus, even if formal aid funding were to increase, it might still not meet all financial needs. Aid offers a much-needed lifeline for the most threatened but continues to leave populations vulnerable to economic shocks, like rising food prices, devalued currency, or, of course, a global pandemic.

In the United States, the limits to our investment in aid and diplomacy are made clear in our budgeting. In 2020, Lockheed Martin, just one arms manufacturer, received $75 billion in government contracts; that is nearly twice as much as the budgets of the entire US State Department and the United States' largest development and humanitarian agency, USAID ($40 billion) (Hartung, 2022). Despite all the money spent on the weapons that are used to wage war, and all the trade that continues to be conducted with countries actively engaging in human rights violations, when it comes to supporting the populations left behind, we can't ever seem to meet our already insufficient fundraising goals.

IT'S TOO INCONSISTENT

The Palestinians received an estimated $37.2 billion in aid from 1994 to 2017. About $9 billion of those funds came from the United States. In fact, the mid-90s saw a significant increase in aid to Palestinians, as external entities wanted to financially support the Oslo Accords and the supposed two-state solution. When Mahmoud Abbas, a politician seen as friendly to the West, was elected president of the Palestinian Authority in the early 2000s, aid increased. When Hamas, a political party considered a terrorist group by the West, won elections in Gaza in 2007, aid dipped. When Democrat Barack Obama won the US presidency in 2008, aid significantly increased, only to fall again in 2012. Global contributions increased the following year by nearly $100 million, but in 2015 they fell to their lowest levels in nearly a decade (World Bank, 2021). Shortly after Republican Donald Trump, who was openly pro-Israel, was elected, he cut US aid to Palestinians significantly, including ending all support to the UNRWA, the UN agency that supports Palestinian refugees. (Previously, the United States was the UNRWA's largest donor.) In 2021, however, newly elected Democratic president Joe Biden reinstated much of the aid to the agency from the United States. Although the aid has changed significantly on a year-to-year basis, the needs on the ground have not. This has been one of the longest and most predictably deteriorating conflicts of the last century. Poverty and food insecurity remain high, unemployment is rising, and a meaningful political resolution seems further away than ever before. Can any population make meaningful development gains with such wild fluctuations in aid?

The unpredictability of aid has long been critiqued in the academic literature about development and state fragility. Some argue that volatility is inherent in humanitarian aid; after all, aid pledges are usually based on unpredictable crisis situations. Often, recipient states are criticized for not making large enough gains when they are provided millions or billions of dollars in aid. When criticizing aid, there are a lot of fair points to make that have been addressed in many studies and books: corruption, inefficiency, and lack of capacity, to name a few. But even the most well-intentioned recipients are doomed to fail. How can a state make a sustainable development plan when it isn't sure what its funding will look like in a year, let alone in five or ten years? Even if donors pledge certain amounts, it's not likely that the recipient will receive the full amount; and recipients don't know just how much or how little they will actually receive or when they'll receive it. This volatility does not just limit meaningful growth but leads to significant waste; one study found that between one-fifth and one-third of aid is wasted due to unpredictability (Kodama, 2011).

While health and education are among the least volatile aid sectors, these needs are often met with short-term initiatives. Much of the most volatile aid is invested in more long-term projects, like those related to industry, government, and program assistance. Health and education, of course, are at the center of many global development efforts, but how we approach outcomes in these sectors is dependent on the type of aid provided (Hudson, 2015). There is a big difference between health aid that leads to a short-term benefit (e.g., a polio vaccination campaign) and aid that leads to a more long-term benefit (e.g., investment in infrastructure that promotes a more functional health system). Because aid is so unpredictable and dispersed at random points of the year, it is much easier to coordinate the former. While these projects are important, they ultimately don't build capacity, as opposed to the long-term projects that will increase societal resilience and health outcomes for years to come. Unless it is transformative, aid is only capable of sustaining a population, at best. But it can't be transformative if it isn't dependable.

IT'S TOO POLITICAL

"Aid is not a gift. The United States provides foreign assistance because it serves our interests and failure is not an option." These were the words of Congressman Howard Berman, then-Ranking Democrat on the House Foreign Affairs Committee, in 2011. While there are many similar quotes from government officials around the world, the bluntness of this one seems particularly telling. Aid is not, in fact, charity, in that it is not merely meant to help those in need in an equitable way. Foreign aid, including that used for humanitarian purposes, is seen by governments as a political tool just like any other. Money earmarked for aid purposes is limited, and how and where that money is dispersed is almost entirely indicative of political goals and not necessarily which populations are most needy. In the United Kingdom, for example, where the aid budget is a mere 0.7% of the gross national income (still one of the highest percentages among wealthy countries), former Prime Minister Theresa May made clear that, "I am unashamed about the need to ensure that our aid programme works for the UK" (Sabbagh, 2018). In fact, none of the world's poorest countries are the top recipients of aid from either the United States or the United Kingdom. Most aid recipients are selected for reasons of politics and, importantly, trade. The top recipient of US aid since 1971, at more than $240 billion, is not Afghanistan, Iraq, Vietnam, or any of the other countries that have suffered as a result of wars instigated by the United States. It is Israel, one of the world's wealthiest and most highly developed countries (Hubbard, 2021).

So, who's lucky enough to get aid? It depends on who's giving it. Some donors, like the Nordic countries, do practice a more needs-based approach to aid. Those with a more recent history of colonialism, like France, Belgium, and Portugal, are more likely to give to former colonies, while the United States has been heavily focused on advancing its aims in the Middle East and has thus spent heavily there (Alesina & Dollar, 2000). When Russia invaded Ukraine in 2022, a worldwide outpouring of aid—to the tune of nearly $100 billion—came within months to help this fledgling nation "in the heart of Europe" counter what was widely seen as unacceptable Russian aggression. To that end, much of it came in the form of military aid—only $8.5 billion was designated for humanitarian funding (Ainsworth, 2022). This demonstrates that it is not just the characteristics of the recipient country that guides how and to where aid is delivered. A large chunk of foreign aid is meant to be spent buying goods or services, including arms, from the donor state, which is beneficial for industry in that country but does too little to build capacity in the crisis-affected country that needs it. In 2017, to defend against calls to cut aid, former USAID administrator Raj Shah confirmed that, "Most U.S. foreign assistance no longer even goes to foreign governments; it is given to U.S. companies and nonprofits in the form of contracts and grants"

(Gerson & Shah, 2017). Although some of these companies and nonprofits may indeed be doing good work on foreign soil, this definition of "foreign assistance" does little to center the needs of the people needing the assistance.

Additionally, evidence suggests that aid is sometimes used as outright leverage against the recipient states. The United States has for decades tied aid to amenable votes at the United Nations. Research shows that more than 70% of aid from the United States goes to countries that agree with the United States, especially when that country rotates into the Security Council and there is a potentially contentious issue to be addressed. Funding from the World Bank, in which the United States plays a key role, follows the same pattern: align with the US position, and you'll be rewarded (Rose, 2018). With such overt political motivations, we can't look at aid as charity, even if many of the individuals who donate to or work within these organizations have charitable intentions. Unless aid is distributed equitably (those who need more receive more), every choice made—where resources are going, how long they will be there, who they will help and how—reflects the priorities and, ultimately, the politics, of the donor country.

DOES HUMANITARIAN AID HELP RECIPIENT NATIONS?

Aside from the above limitations, there are other reasons to question whether outsourcing support for needy populations should be centered around providing them aid. Aid effectiveness has been a hot topic in the development and humanitarian sectors for several decades. It seems apparent that in times of absolute crisis—a tsunami, an outbreak of polio, a refugee crisis—a rapid influx of external support, utilized well, can absolutely prevent widespread suffering and chaos. But there are a lot of variables involved in ensuring that happens; and remember, most of our modern crises are not acute and temporary but protracted and extremely complex. How does aid function in that environment? A lot of research has shown that aid entrenches dependence (some have referred to it as neocolonialism), often ignores the needs of local people by focusing on donor priorities, and doesn't contribute to long-term development that would increase outcomes in a meaningful and sustainable way. Some have even argued that aid can prolong conflicts, support warmongers, and have disastrous effects on local currencies and markets.

I'm not arguing to abolish aid. Without a massive political and economic shift in the global approach to war, aid is necessary. With increasing natural disasters from climate change in the coming century, aid is going to be even more necessary. I know many wonderful and deserving people whose lives have benefited from humanitarian aid, whether in the form of a scholarship, a meal, a loan, a health care procedure, a phone, or a vaccine. However, for every surgery that is paid for and every meal that is distributed, there are dozens more people in need of medical care or food that are not sufficiently helped. Further, as conflicts continue, the need for more medical care and more food continues to increase.

Aid does indeed fill gaps that would otherwise go unfilled. However, it does little about the reasons those gaps are unfilled to begin with. Again, it's not meant to! The problem is not necessarily with the aid itself but with what the aid is expected to do. Too often, aid is used as a cushion to avoid addressing root causes of conflicts by offering only humanitarian solutions to inherently political problems. Or, worse, it is used as a tool to benefit parties outside of the affected populations—sometimes, the donor itself, through serving their political or economic goals. It's hard to think of anything more cynical than providing goods and services to needy people while pushing political or military aims that don't ultimately benefit those people or may even actively harm them.

It feels good to help people who need it. Opinion polls from many donor countries show that populations generally support providing aid (even if they vastly overestimate just how much aid is being given). But what would genuinely benefit conflict-affected populations is to help them gain safety, stability, and full recognition of their human rights. Aid is not meant to do that. Aid *cannot* do that. And so instead of looking at aid as a response to war, we should see it as almost a completely distinct and parallel process; it happens during and around war and other crises, but it has little to do with ending them. While providing aid to needy people, the goal should be to use every political and economic lever to ensure that aid provision does not need to last for years or decades and that it sincerely addresses the reason the aid is needed to begin with. Instead, we use aid to avoid having to pull the political and economic levers that are uncomfortable or controversial, even if that means prolonging the suffering altogether and causing demand for aid that we're unwilling to fully meet.

Yes, aid should be there to pull people out of immediate danger when it's unavoidable. But building schools and hospitals should be the job of responsive and inclusive governments, not foreign donors, no matter how well-intentioned. Aid agencies, especially the large multinational ones, are not accountable to affected populations but to their donors and other stakeholders. In the best case, sometimes they will get input from local populations or partner with community groups. When they do, they better incorporate local contexts and cultures, they develop ownership of programming in local communities, they build local capacity, and they can access populations that are remote or would otherwise be overlooked; importantly, they enable accountability mechanisms for populations affected by humanitarian efforts (OECD, 2017). Unfortunately, however, they too frequently don't, or they only do so on a superficial level. Regardless, war-affected people don't want or need endless handouts. They need the end of war.

REFERENCES

Ainsworth, D. (2022, August 22). Funding tracker: Who's sending aid to Ukraine? Devex.

Alesina, A., & Dollar, D. (2000). Who gives foreign aid to whom and why? *Journal of Economic Growth, 5*, 33–63.

Clarke, K. (2018). *The state of the humanitarian system 2018—full report.* ALNAP. https://www.alnap.org/system/files/content/resource/files/main/SOHS%20Online%20Book%201%20updated.pdf.

Development Initiatives. (2020). *Global humanitarian assistance report 2020.* https://devinit.org/documents/776/Global-Humanitarian-Assistance-Report-2020.pdf.

Gerson, M., & Shah, R. (2017, February 24). "America first" shouldn't mean cutting foreign aid. *The Washington Post.* https://www.washingtonpost.com/posteverything/wp/2017/02/24/america-first-shouldnt-mean-cutting-foreign-aid/.

Hartung, W. (2022). How private contractors disguise the real costs of war. *Inkstick Media.* https://inkstickmedia.com/how-private-contractors-disguise-the-real-costs-of-war/.

House Foreign Affairs Committee. (2011). *Congressman Howard Berman releases discussion draft of foreign assistance reform plan.* https://democrats-foreignaffairs.house.gov/press-releases?ID=894962B3-1DAA-4F51-8ED4-0D089AACF0E7.

Hubbard, K. (2021, May 24). 3 charts that illustrate where U.S. foreign aid goes. *U.S. News & World Report.* https://www.usnews.com/news/best-countries/articles/2021-05-24/afghanistan-israel-largest-recipients-of-us-foreign-aid.

Hudson, J. (2015). Consequences of aid volatility for macroeconomic management and aid effectiveness. *World Development, 69*, 62–74.

Kodama, M. (2011). Aid unpredictability and economic growth. *World Development, 40*(2), 266–272.

Organisation for Economic Co-operation and Development (OECD). (2017). *Localising the response.* https://www.oecd.org/development/humanitarian-donors/docs/Localisingtheresponse.pdf.

Organisation for Economic Co-operation and Development (OECD). (2019). *Lives in crises: What do people tell us about the humanitarian aid they receive?* https://doi.org/10.1787/9d39623d-en.

Rose, S. (2018). *Linking US foreign aid to UN votes: What are the implications?* Center for Global Development. https://www.cgdev.org/publication/linking-us-foreign-aid-un-votes-what-are-implications.

Sabbagh, D. (2018, August 27). May begins Africa trip with nod to rightwing Tories on overseas aid. *The Guardian.* https://www.theguardian.com/politics/2018/aug/27/may-africa-trip-rightwing-tories-overseas-aid.

United Nations. (2021a, February 17). *Food insecurity in Syria reaches record levels: WFP.* https://news.un.org/en/story/2021/02/1084972#.

United Nations. (2021b, March 30). *As plight of Syrians worsens, hunger reaches record high, international community must fully commit to ending decade-old war, secretary-general tells General Assembly.* https://www.un.org/press/en/2021/sgsm20664.doc.htm.

United Nations. (2021c, September 19). *COVID vaccines: Widening inequality and millions vulnerable.* https://news.un.org/en/story/2021/09/1100192.

World Bank. (2021). *Net ODA received per capita (current US$)—West Bank and Gaza.* https://data.worldbank.org/indicator/DT.ODA.ODAT.PC.ZS?locations=PS.

World Food Programme (WFP). (2021). *Twelve million Syrians now in the grip of hunger, worn down by conflict and soaring food prices.* https://www.wfp.org/news/twelve-million-syrians-now-grip-hunger-worn-down-conflict-and-soaring-food-prices.

CONCLUSION

Now I want to deal with the third evil that constitutes the dilemma of our nation and the world. And that is the evil of war. Somehow these three evils are tied together. The triple evils of racism, economic exploitation, and militarism. The great problem and the great challenge facing mankind today is to get rid of war. . . . During a period of war, when a nation becomes obsessed with the guns of war, social programs inevitably suffer. People become insensitive to pain and agony in their own midst . . .

Now I know that there are people who are confused about the war and they say to me and anybody who speaks out against it, "You shouldn't be speaking out. You're a civil rights leader, and the two issues should not be joined together." Well . . . the two issues are tied together. And I'm going to keep them together. Oh my friends, it's good for us to fight for integrated lunch counters, and for integrated schools. And I'm going to continue to do that. But wouldn't it be absurd to be talking about integrated schools without being concerned about the survival of a world in which to be integrated . . .

—DR. MARTIN LUTHER KING JR., in an address to the Hungry Club Forum (1967)

The tyrant will always find a pretext for his tyranny, and it is useless for the innocent to try by reasoning to get justice, when the oppressor intends to be unjust.

—AESOP, "The Wolf and the Lamb" (sixth century BCE)

DURING THE SPANISH CIVIL WAR in the 1930s, planes from the fascist Italian and Nazi German regimes bombed the Spanish city of Guernica, in part to allow for a ground invasion by General Francisco Franco and his Nationalist forces. The attack, called Operation Rügen, targeted the town because of its position as the last town to conquer before Franco could capture Bilbao, the capital of the Basque Country. There were no military targets in the town; the attack was specifically directed at civilians and was conducted on a Monday, a market day, when the attack's perpetrators were sure many people would be out of their homes. The attack horrified the world, including a Spanish painter named Pablo Picasso, who would go on to produce the painting *Guernica* within months of the attack, which is now recognized as one of his greatest works and even one of the greatest works of art in history. While representative of Picasso's abstract style, the pain in the painting is clear; there are limbs scattered throughout the scene, what appears to be a woman wailing as she clutches a dead baby, and a man painted in utter distress, being swallowed by the violence of war. Today, a replica of the piece is hung in the United Nations headquarters in New York City.

A few years later in 1941, another Spanish artist, Salvador Dali, painted *The Face of War*, also inspired by the horrors of the Spanish Civil War. More than a century before, Francisco Goya created a series of prints, *The Disasters of War*, about the ugliness of an entirely different war in Spain. Artists from across cultures and across time have tried to express the truth about war where words often fail. Look at *The War Series* by Käthe Kollwitz; *We Shall Return* by Imad Abu Shtayyah; *The Apotheosis of War* by Vasily Vereshchagin; or *Soldiers Playing Cards* by Fernand Léger and try not to feel something—often, something uncomfortable.

You don't have to be a fan of paintings, of course, to see how society and culture view war and militarization—and we don't even have to consider the countless movies and TV shows directly related to war, although there are many. (*M*A*S*H*, a show about an army field hospital during the Korean War, is considered one of the greatest American TV shows of all time. And movies like *All Quiet on the Western Front*, *Dr. Strangelove*, *Schindler's List*, *Saving Private Ryan*, and *Full Metal Jacket* are regarded as staples of American cinema.) Forrest Gump's beloved partner, Lieutenant Dan, suffered extreme PTSD after losing his legs in the Vietnam War. The protagonist of the TV show *WandaVision* realizes her extraordinary powers after a bomb falls on her apartment, killing her parents and traumatizing her and her younger brother. The entire premise of the movie *Jurassic World: Fallen Kingdom* is centered around arms dealers who figure out how to manufacture a dinosaur that is essentially an indestructible weapon and sell it on the black market. In 2015, a play called *Grounded* portrayed the increasing mental distress of a female Air Force pilot safely living in Las Vegas but using drones to bomb Afghanistan. And who could forget the war references in songs like "Zombie" by the Cranberries, "Gimme Shelter" by the Rolling Stones, and even "1999" by Prince. The recognition that war is often unjust, destructive, and ultimately futile permeates every aspect of our culture. But we persist in justifying it or trusting those who do.

The purpose of this book is certainly not to convince anyone that war is bad. I believe that almost everyone already believes that. However, I do want to convince you that war is not, as we're too often led to believe, inevitable, or even beneficial, most of the time. It's *not* too complex to understand and have opinions about. It's not just bad for the people that live in it; it's bad for you too. You don't need access to classified security documents, a job at a prominent think tank or university, or a history degree (or any degree) to understand this. These are distractions from the reality, which is what you can plainly see and already intrinsically understand. Bombing civilians? It's bad. It doesn't matter if the person doing it wears a uniform, even if it's a uniform bearing the flag of the country you're from. It doesn't even matter if it's an accident. If you have the power to launch a missile out of a plane onto foreign land, you should be fully prepared to accept every potential outcome and be willing to be held accountable for any of them. And if a few accidental bombings happen, all the time, with no one getting in trouble, and global injustices persist no matter how many trillions we throw at militaries and arms manufacturers—and the stakeholders benefitting from war are, when we think about it, not exactly who we want to put on a pedestal at the center of society—it seems kind of crazy that this, of all political conversations, is the one that is supposed to be open and shut. We simply must have the strongest military . . . don't we? We absolutely have to threaten others to get what we want, obviously, and what we want is always the right outcome for everyone, even if they don't know it yet, right? We wouldn't accept this posture in any other sector, but the one that has the power and legal standing to literally kill others is offered the greatest protection and afforded the luxury of ignoring self-reflection and accountability. We don't have the time for self-reflection, hippie! Lock and load.

War and the industries, philosophies, and interests that support it are the biggest threat to the health and well-being of all people. As conducted today, war is, indeed, an epidemic of modern times. But epidemics can and do end. I recognize the folly of calling for an immediate end to all war and forms of militarism. There are too many interests, too many egos, and too few incentives for those that engage in the war industry. Many people implicitly support war without really knowing why; that's how normalized the acceptance of war and violence has become. These beliefs became entrenched somehow. And so there must be mechanisms with which to unwind and rethink our approach to peace and conflict. There have been many books and articles written about ending war and alternatives to war, and it is impossible to do justice to such a multifaceted concept in one chapter. Instead, what I hope to do is present a range of ways to think differently that can start to pry open our assumptions of war, what it means, and if we really need it.

RETHINKING THE MEANING OF SECURITY

What is the definition of "national security"? Think about it for a moment. It probably brings to mind some idea of a nation's ability to protect its borders from external threats, primarily through military might, with a bit of diplomacy or economic leverage thrown in for good measure. Now, nobody wants their country attacked; and, if attacked, most people would support some measure of retaliation. They might even expect it. One of the primary functions of a state is to protect its citizens from such external threats, and it's a fair expectation. But this has led to an overt dependence on militarization as the primary source of security, with every other aspect of life essentially getting whatever crumbs are left over.

Yet, who is really feeling secure these days? Do Americans, with the most powerful and dominant military humankind has ever seen, really feel secure? Do parents feel secure when dropping their children off at school, hoping it isn't the day a mass shooter comes to campus? Do politicians feel secure entering their workplace, knowing a kidnapping plot or insurrection is one potential Facebook post away? Do we feel secure when apartment buildings burn down due to a faulty space heater because tenants had no access to heating? Can anyone feel secure knowing a factory is pumping toxins into their local air or water, whether they're in Cambodia or Texas? Does it make us feel secure knowing that grocery stores and restaurants throw away literal tons of food every day while many of our fellow citizens go hungry? Does the development of a new F-35 jet, estimated to cost $1.5 trillion over its lifespan—that quite literally burst into flames on the tarmac during testing and still reports dozens of operational errors even as it goes into mass production—make anyone feel safer or more protected? And who feels secure in the richest country in history when it cannot reasonably handle a (hopefully) once-in-a-generation pandemic while the wealthiest people in the country got even richer than they'd been the year before and were able to take their private jets to secluded islands while the rest of us sat home and washed our groceries?

In a groundbreaking report often cited by humanitarians and academics but seemingly ignored by everyone else, the United Nations attempted to redefine security in 1994 (United Nations, 1994). They conceptualized the idea of *human security*, which, instead of being based around the security of the state (national security) was centered around the security of people. Human security includes political security but must not end there. It considers economic security, food security, health security, environmental security, personal security, and community security to be forms of security necessary to support not just survival but the ability to thrive. The report defines this multifaceted form of security as universal (relevant to all people, everywhere) and interdependent. Human security emphasizes prevention over intervention, which is cheaper and averts many of these threats to national security from developing in the first place (United Nations, 1994).

In the report, they point out that many of the world's poorest countries spend more on their military than on health and education. The authors also recognize that insecurity in any of the aforementioned sectors is, in fact, more likely to lead to conflict, deprivation, and, in turn, a greater emphasis on the security offered by militaries, leading to a vicious cycle. This premise of militarization as the ultimate goal of governments is simply not working. Again, this report was released nearly 30 years ago, and the loose concept of human security existed long before that. Just imagine what today might look like if this approach to security had been adopted. It's not too late to do so.

ENFORCING ACCOUNTABILITY MECHANISMS

We have many laws, conventions, tribunals, treaties, and agreements that are meant to protect the vulnerable and prosecute the powerful. We have multiple international organizations and alliances, even an International Criminal Court, that were developed with heady goals of preventing atrocities and holding perpetrators accountable. Yet our collective willingness to not rock the boat, to prioritize economic partnerships and capitalist values over our own stated ethics and principles, to trust that all elites have good intentions despite overwhelming evidence to the contrary, and to hold our allies, and ourselves, to different standards than we hold our enemies, have hollowed out the meaning of many of these agreements and organizations.

Just a few chapters ago, I discussed the disastrous drone strike conducted by the United States shortly after the withdrawal from Afghanistan that killed 10 Afghani civilians. A few months later, after a "high-level" investigation, the Pentagon concluded that there were "no violations of law" and that any disciplinary action against those involved should be left to military commanders. You'll be shocked to know that those commanders decided not to punish anyone and that the defense secretary agreed (Schmitt, 2021). Let's remember that the military called this a legitimate strike until a *New York Times* investigation found otherwise (Koettl et al., 2021). So that's it. Ten people killed, most of whom were children, by drones funded by the American taxpayer, and not a single person was held accountable. And this happens over, and over, and over again.

In December 2021, the *New York Times* released another bombshell report, meticulously reporting that throughout the so-called War on Terror, through Democratic and Republican administrations, the US military killed thousands of civilians, primarily through airstrikes (Khan, 2021). Instead of any form of public reckoning, apology, reparations, or even a fundamental rethinking of what former President Obama called "the most precise air campaign in history," the US military ignored and sidelined analysts who warned about risks to civilians, hid or classified reports containing evidence of such attacks, and deemed eyewitness reports of civilian casualties to be uncredible. Also in 2021, Daniel Hale, a former US intelligence analyst who leaked classified information about the drone program to a reporter after learning of how flawed the operations were (including classifying all military-aged males as "enemies killed in action" no matter what they were doing or who they were), was sentenced to 45 months in prison. We definitely know how to hold people accountable when we want to, it seems.

Lack of accountability is not limited to the United States, of course. The ongoing bombing campaign of Yemen by Saudi Arabia, often with American-made weapons, has been criticized by some politicians but continues to be funded. This is the same Saudi government that the United States claimed it was sure had ordered the assassination of journalist Jamal Khashoggi and the same Saudi government that has imprisoned women for driving and bloggers for criticizing the monarchy. Despite this, the Saudi foreign minister had a "great meeting" with American Secretary of State Antony Blinken in July 2021, who just months earlier pledged to put human rights "at the center of US foreign policy" (US Department of State, 2021). Israel has long been criticized for decades of human rights violations, including an ongoing military occupation, a separation wall deemed illegal by the International Court of Justice, continued settlement expansion, overt reliance on extrajudicial killings and administrative detentions, and massive bombing campaigns that kill hundreds and sometimes thousands of civilians (again, often with American weapons). In 2019, the US government signed yet another military aid pledge to the nation, appropriating $38 billion to Israel from just 2019–2028. China is accused of detaining up to a million religious and ethnic minorities in internment camps in Xinjiang, where Tesla recently opened a fabulous new showroom. Despite multiple other well-documented human rights violations, China also maintained the honor of hosting the 2022 Winter Olympics.

The UN Security Council has attempted to pass multiple resolutions on Syria, all blocked by Russia, which happened to be actively engaged in bombing the country. In 2021, several Arab states reopened communication with Syria's President Bashar al-Assad, notwithstanding the last 10 years of his military bombing the country into utter destruction and being responsible for the deaths or disappearances of hundreds of thousands of Syrians. Despite being well known for bombing hospitals, blocking convoys of aid, using chemical weapons, and murdering and detaining countless health workers, Syria was elected to the World Health Organization Executive Board in 2021. Egypt, a country that receives more than $1 billion in military aid from the United States annually, has one of the worst human rights records in modern times, which includes the jailing of up to 60,000 political prisoners. Under President Rodrigo Duterte, the Philippines engaged in an unprecedented campaign of extrajudicial killings and other human rights violations. But in 2021, the United States affirmed there would be "no restrictions" on arms sales to this purported ally. The list goes on and on. With friends like these . . .

It's simple: we cannot end war if we do not end impunity. And this doesn't mean holding accountable just the individual actors who perpetrate crimes, but also the systems and leadership that enable and encourage them to do so. This wouldn't necessarily require any kind of shake-up in international law; we have many appropriate mechanisms for investigating and prosecuting perpetrators of human rights violations. Unfortunately, the power to end impunity largely rests with the entities with significant interests in maintaining it. When evidence of potential crimes is so overwhelming that investigations become inevitable, governments and militaries usually conduct their own secret investigations and, unsurprisingly, almost always find no fault. Often, they'll blame process errors or even cynically use claims of self-defense, no matter how egregious or preemptive the action. Victims and their families have almost no recourse for lost lives or property and instead are often blamed for being "human shields" or just considered "collateral damage." In 2020, an Iraqi man made global headlines for being the first civilian to be compensated for an airstrike during the War on Terror. US intelligence mistakenly identified the home of Basim Razzo as an ISIS headquarters, and a Dutch F-16 jet launched a "precision strike" on the area, killing his wife, daughter, brother, and nephew and rendering Razzo unable to walk. The Dutch government decided to "voluntarily" offer him nearly €1 million, while still "not admitting liability over the deaths" (Boffey, 2020).

Even the International Criminal Court (ICC), established in 2002 to investigate and prosecute war crimes and crimes against humanity, lacks authority, faces significant bureaucratic obstacles to investigation, is highly politicized, and doesn't have the support of several of the world's most powerful states (China, Russia, and the United States aren't even members of the ICC). Militaries and defense contractors are rarely held accountable for loss and waste in budgets, let alone loss of life. Global corruption—including nepotism, clientelism, bribery, patronage, grift, and tax evasion—is rampant and widely accepted, even when the losses are obvious and significant. If it sounds like I'm wading too much into political science here, consider how the money and trust lost to corruption impacts health. In 2003, for example, the United States spent more than $100 million to build Basra's Children's Hospital in Iraq, meant to be a world-class hospital for children with cancer. The hospital opened in 2011, six years behind schedule, and corruption in the form of skimming, inflated contracts, overpriced goods, extortion, and money that just plain disappeared has essentially reduced the hospital to a waiting room for sick children. There aren't even enough chairs for parents to sit in as they await diagnoses for their children, often of ailments the hospital isn't equipped to treat (Loveluck & Salim, 2021). Instead of accountability, we might get some hearings, committees, white papers, and reports that go nowhere, if there is any action at all, almost ensuring future violations.

CHALLENGING THE ROLE OF THE ARMS INDUSTRY

Every industry, from fossil fuels to processed foods to fast fashion, has its problems. But the arms industry is unlike any other. Unlike the goods that have everyday uses that are produced by most other industries, weapons have no use in the absence of violence. The idea that weapons and other military-grade materials should be commodities that are bought and sold like any other should be called out for the misguided and naïve assumption that history has shown us time and time again that it is. Universities, 401(k)s, retirement accounts, pension plans, and index funds have billions invested in arms manufacturers (Evans & Behar, 2018). Arms sales are used as political levers without a second thought. Tobacco companies needed people to smoke and chew tobacco to keep their businesses afloat; that's just how business works. They had every incentive to keep their industry going; and they did, despite their own internal knowledge that their product was harmful, even lethal. Why would one country provide weapons to another if they didn't have the expectation that they would be used, even if just to intimidate another country? Is this the best use of the energy, influence, and power of the United States as the world's main arms manufacturer, and its political and economic prowess?

It may be unrealistic to hope for a day where there is no need for weaponry or an arms industry. Use of this point by proponents of the industry is meant to shut down any discussion of limiting or restricting arms sales, especially to foreign entities. However, what is stopping well-intentioned countries from banning the sale of weapons or provision of military support to countries that are actively engaged in conflict or have engaged in war crimes, at a bare minimum? Can't we at least engage in conversations about divestment from arms manufacturers, regulation, and even accountability regarding how weapons are ultimately used? Limiting weapons will not end war; it is possible to harm many people with forms of structural violence. But it will end suffering for a lot of people, and that's a start.

LINKING WAR AND MILITARISM TO HEALTH AND WELL-BEING

Despite my best efforts, it's impossible to account for all the links between war and health in one book. Not just because no one book could cover it all, but because there is a severe lack of research on so many of the different ways war and militarism interact with human health or limit our ability to manage health and other aspects of well-being.

In the United States, research about the effects of gun violence on public health was basically banned for 20 years, for essentially one reason: some people in power didn't want to know or didn't want what they suspected was true to become publicly known. If you know, then it's harder to pretend something is not a problem. Best to ignore the phenomena entirely and consider those who call for research or investigation "partisans." For example, when more than 200,000 soldiers who had returned from Iraq started complaining about breathing problems and other respiratory ailments due to burn pits, the Department of Veterans Affairs discouraged or even censored reports from doctors describing the ailments while at the same time denying burn-pit exposure claims from veterans due to a lack of conclusive data (Stack, 2022). (Speaking of accountability, the private contractor that ran the burn pits, KBR, fought lawsuits so they could avoid paying damages to soldiers; in 2019, the Supreme Court decided that private contractors were immune to such lawsuits, citing the same rulings that protect the military's decisions.) Importantly, doctors and researchers are typically seen as credible, nonpartisan witnesses. If they come to conclusions blaming certain actors for negative health effects, well, that could become quite messy—and expensive.

I think this purposeful ignorance is part of the reason the study of war is not adequately supported, but it's not the only reason. Conducting research on war is difficult and can be expensive, especially research that requires access to dangerous environments. Fragile populations are hard to reach or may fear being honest with researchers, especially with foreigners they don't know or in countries with harsh penalties for dissent. Wars can start up quickly, which doesn't give researchers time to secure funding (which is limited) or permissions (which require a lot of ethical considerations for working with fragile populations). Since war usually occurs in low- and middle-income countries where data collection may already be limited, it's hard to conduct longitudinal studies that track specific data points over time. Linking one specific phenomenon—war—with health outcomes is also difficult. How do we parse the effects of war when there are so many threats to health that are related to war but are not limited to the war environment, like poverty, gender inequality, food insecurity, and poor health infrastructure? On top of that, many public health programs and medical schools don't teach about war or militarism—they are seen as niche topics in global health at best, and you're lucky to find a graduate seminar on the topic at most universities.

Because of the gap between how we look at health and how we think of war, we tend to think of war as the domain of political scientists and economists, not of health researchers or practitioners. But, as I hope I've demonstrated throughout this book, war is fundamentally a threat to health, directly and indirectly. Health researchers should give war the same consideration they've given to any other threat to health, like smoking, drinking, homelessness, racism, gun violence, or climate change. War should be considered a social determinant of health, just like education, employment, and housing, and studied as such. Scholars in disciplines outside of health should more readily integrate evidence about the human consequences of conflict into their assessments, while all scholars should recognize the ways militarism shapes our cultures and limits the imagination in terms of what is possible in dealing with any number of issues. And the media plays a part here, too. Journalists are not meant to blindly repeat the talking points of a government, especially one that was just accused of doing something terribly wrong. The media has the job of observing and interpreting complex societal trends, like militarism, which it rarely does. It is understandable that the average person in a stable country may not connect the dots between war and their own lives, but it is not understandable that the media does not help them do so.

QUESTIONING THE JUSTIFICATIONS FOR WAR

Despite movies and video games, war is, thankfully, an abstract concept to most. Not just because people don't witness it with their own eyes—we've all seen the news, and videos direct from war zones are easy to find on social media these days—but because the horror is often too much for our minds to meaningfully process. We hear the numbers of the dead and injured, and sometimes a video or photo will make its way around social media. Yet the everyday brutal reality of what war does to people is largely hidden from the public because it serves as evidence of what warfare actually looks like—not ticker-tape parades brimming with flag-waving and proud families, not soldiers "greeted as liberators" by newly democratized populations, but dead children, destroyed hospitals, and starving elders. This isn't the allied forces valiantly fighting the Nazis; these are wars that most people don't understand and can't explain. Why are US soldiers dying in Niger? Why is Saudi Arabia bombing Yemen, and why is the United States okay with it? Was there really a near-genocide against the Rohingya and no one really did anything about it? You shouldn't need a PhD in international relations to explain why your country is at war with one country and not intervening in another; and when you feel like you do, it is easy to disconnect, turn off the TV or close the web browser, and hope for the best.

Don't we, at some point, have to ask if wars are justified in their aims? Are drone attacks, airstrikes, or sieges successful in any long-term capacity regarding political goals? Are nonlethal weapons actually successful in safely dispersing crowds—and are they really "nonlethal" at all? Does assassinating the leader of a militant organization actually lead to positive outcomes in the long run? Is "collateral damage" truly unavoidable, with no long-term negative impacts on strategic goals? We are told to just assume that the answer to all these questions is yes, despite evidence to the contrary. In fact, there are dozens of studies that show that war, as currently practiced, is rarely effective in achieving its initial goals. Often what happens is a war is waged, it destabilizes a country or region, and then the justifications for the war shift to deal with that destabilization. The initial reason is often forgotten, and no one has to answer for it. The fog of war, right? But at that point, we're in too deep to simply pull out and admit failure.

The field of peace research has had to find ways to quantify and justify peace and incorporate peacebuilding into economic and development programming (rather than let peace be a goal in and of itself), but peace research remains marginalized. Meanwhile, those advocating for war are never called to prove their claims, despite how many thousands of these claims are later proven incorrect and, in many cases, are actively covered up and lied about until some shred of evidence is uncovered. The answer to terrorists is to have bigger bombs and inhumane prisons; the answer to fear is larger military budgets; the answer to war is more war. But these assumptions expect us to collectively ignore what we intrinsically know: Replacing weapons with supposedly nonlethal weapons isn't revolutionary; drones are not humane; airstrikes are not precise. War is not peace; war is just violent, ugly, brutal war.

CLOSING THOUGHT

"War is over if you want it." So go the lyrics of the song "Happy Xmas (War Is Over)" by John Lennon and Yoko Ono. Maybe it's just a silly little song by two of America's most famous peace activists, a couple of hippies deeply embedded in the counterculture calling for an end to the Vietnam War. What an ugly war that was. And what an ugly war they all are. That's the thing: they're all ugly. There are few winners in war that are actually *in* the war. Most of the winners are safely tucked away in capitals and boardrooms, making decisions that don't affect them about the lives of people they don't recognize.

Maybe it's not just a lyric though. Just over three years into the COVID-19 pandemic, the head of the World Health Organization declared an end to COVID-19 as a public health emergency (while still cautioning that, "It is still killing and it is still changing."). But the war epidemic is thousands of years in the making, and there seems to be no end in sight. Don't we—all of us—deserve better? But for a stroke of fate, it could be our child washed up on the shore, our mother who needs chemotherapy in a country with no hospital, our spouse who is picked up by the authorities one day and never returns. If we continue into this spiral of militarism, we are bringing ourselves closer to that reality, not further away. Where do we think this ends? Does anyone really believe that war brings peace anymore? Violence begets more violence, as it always has, and feeding the war machine doesn't satiate it. It only grows bigger and demands more. But war can be over, as John and Yoko might say, if we want it.

Many of us value our health and the health of our loved ones above anything else. Yet we sacrifice bits of our health and well-being every day for the right to live in a country with trillion-dollar jets while at the same time justifying injury and death of others, including of our own vaunted servicepeople. The challenges of the world in the coming century are not going to decrease. We have an aging global population, climate change and parts of the planet that are becoming uninhabitable, democratic backsliding all over the world, rampant misinformation and conspiracy theories made more visible by advances in technology we barely understand, and politicians who are willing to exploit all of it to maintain power. And that's just what we have to worry about as this damn pandemic ends. War and militarism limit our ability to make any progress on these issues or any others. We can, and must, think differently, and most importantly, act differently.

I've spent a lot of time in this book talking about the history of how we got to where we are today. But ultimately, that's all it is: history. "We do not inherit the earth from our ancestors; we borrow it from our children," as the proverb goes. What do we want to leave for our children? What lessons have we learned from centuries of bloodshed and suffering? War is an epidemic. And we must end it.

REFERENCES

Boffey, D. (2020, September 9). Mosul civilian first to be compensated for mistaken coalition bombing. *The Guardian*. https://www.theguardian.com/world

/2020/sep/09/mosul-civilian-first-to-be-compensated-for-mistaken-coal ition-bombing.

Evans, J., & Behar, A. (2018, June 26). Who is making a killing on killing? *Common Dreams.* https://www.commondreams.org/views/2018/06/26/who-making -killing-killing.

Khan, A. (2021, December 18). Hidden Pentagon records reveal patterns of failure in deadly airstrikes. *The New York Times.* https://www.nytimes.com/interactive /2021/12/18/us/airstrikes-pentagon-records-civilian-deaths.html.

Koettl, C., Hill, E., Aikins, M., Schmitt, E., Tiefenthäler, A., & Jordan, D. (2021, September 10). How a U.S. drone strike killed the wrong person. *The New York Times.* https://www.nytimes.com/video/world/asia/100000007963596/us -drone-attack-kabul-investigation.html.

Loveluck, L., & Salim, M. (2021, December 16). The U.S. built a hospital for Iraqi children with cancer. Corruption ravaged it. *The Washington Post.* https://www .washingtonpost.com/world/2021/12/16/iraq-hospital-corruption/.

Schmitt, E. (2021, December 13). No U.S. troops will be punished for deadly Kabul strike, Pentagon chief decides. *The New York Times.* https://www.nytimes .com/2021/12/13/us/politics/afghanistan-drone-strike.html.

Stack, M. (2022, January 11). The soldiers came home sick. The government denied it was responsible. *The New York Times.* https://www.nytimes.com/2022/01 /11/magazine/military-burn-pits.html.

United Nations. (1994). *Human development report 1994.* http://hdr.undp.org /sites/default/files/reports/255/hdr_1994_en_complete_nostats.pdf.

US Department of State. (2021, February 24). *Putting human rights at the center of U.S. foreign policy.* https://www.state.gov/putting-human-rights-at-the-center -of-u-s-foreign-policy/.

INDEX